The Human Pony:
A Guide for Owners, Trainers and Admirers

by Rebecca Wilcox

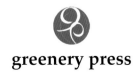

greenery press

Published in the United States by Greenery Press, 4200 Park Blvd. pmb 240, Oakland, CA 94602, www.greenerypress.com.

ISBN 978-1890159-99-3.

Contents

Foreword *by Trigger the Human Equine* v

A Personal Word vii

Introduction xiv

1   **What Is Pony Play?** 1

2.   **Pony and Trainer Headspace** 13

3.   **Equipment** 19

4.   **Training Your Pony** 39

5.   **Scene Development** 53

6.   **Handling and Grooming** 71

7.   **The Inspiration – The Horse** 85

8.   **Event Planning: Do It Yourself** 97

     Conclusion: End on a Good Note 113

     Appendix A: Gaits 115

     Appendix B: Quick Release Knot 125

     Appendix C: Pony Play Glossary 128

     Appendix D: Related Resources 136

     Contributors and Acknowledgments 139

Foreword
by Trigger The Human Equine

I have often been asked, "How did you get into pony play?" And the honest answer is: I owe it all to Elvis Presley.

I was a big Elvis fan in my youth. When Elvis died, it seemed as though his photo was on the cover of every magazine and newspaper I saw. I especially liked the photo on the cover of a magazine I'd never heard of – Penthouse *Variations* – so I bought a copy.

I was a young man, naïve to the ways of the world and utterly clueless about sex and kink. But the first article I read in the magazine was a first-person tale of pony play – and I was hooked.

That was back in the 1970s, and, boy, have I evolved. But I learned the hard way, because at that time there were no pony play handbooks, no webpages (in fact, no Internet), and no support groups or clubs. And telling a typical 1970s woman that I wanted to be ridden as her horse was beyond impossible: they mostly thought that what I wanted was for them to be on top during the kind of sex they were used to, which was not even close to what I had in mind.

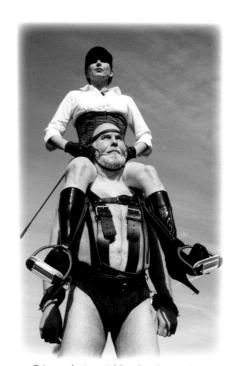

Trigger being ridden by the author.

But I didn't give up. The years passed and I continued my quest for riders who would understand. I finally realized that if I wanted to be a horse, I needed to look the part – I needed a harness, a saddle, a bridle – something to help make my equine self a reality.

In the 1990s I met an understanding leathercrafter who made me my first pony harness. Now all I needed was someone to hold it. I didn't know exactly what I wanted to do once I found her – all I knew was that I wanted to be a horse, and I wanted a woman to ride me. Imagine the thrill when I wore my harness to my first leather event – Diversions, in Florida – and a woman actually came up to me and asked if she could have a ride!

Since that amazing day, I've had over five hundred different riders enjoy everything from a short jaunt of a few minutes to a nice long ride of an hour or more. I've traveled all over the world promoting pony play, and have been involved with TV shows including *HBO Real Sex,* VH1's *Wide World of Online Dating, Playboy Sexcetera,* and *The Tyra Banks Show,* as well as several shows in Europe. There have been more magazine articles and photo spreads than I can count. It's been a great life as a horse.

If, back in the '70s, I could have read the book you now hold in your hands, it could have brought me a decade more pleasure and excitement (as well as sparing me a few embarrassing and upsetting mistakes). But I take comfort in knowing that never again will an excited and fearful young horse-to-be have to be told "I just don't get it" by a potential rider or trainer – because now, anyone with an interest or curiosity about this thrilling kink has a comprehensive and fun-to-read handbook to help them learn, participate, understand, or even just admire the wonderful world of pony play.

Brava Rebecca!!

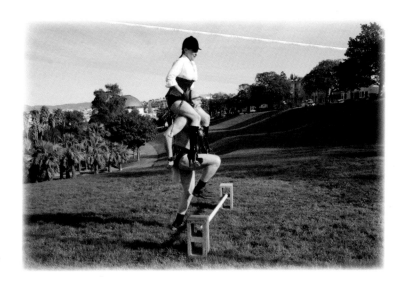

A Personal Word

Although I've been trained in a variety of sports involving horses, my formal equestrian background predominantly features basic English seat and dressage. My experience ranges from my childhood 4-H Club membership to the training of my own Mustang-Hanoverian stallion.

When I first explored my interest in human pony play, there was a marked shortage of trainers. Soon after I began my participation in the leather lifestyle I found a welcome place for my equestrian talents and their natural offshoot, animal role-play. Impassioned to support pony play and pony players through community participation, presentations, workshops and educational materials, I quickly became a pony play activist.

My experience with genetic horses heavily influenced my play and by extension my teaching. Horses are intrinsic to my happiness. Riding in a car seat as a little girl, I yearned for the horses in the field. Deep inside my body a voice screamed, "I want that!" My entire focus as a child revolved around horses: I wanted to own horses, ride horses, groom horses, smell horses and spend every minute of every day at the barn. My parents conceded to let me ride the burros at Knott's Berry Farm, the Southern California tourist attraction, at an early age. Riding and horsemanship lessons began at age eight, in response to the nearly daily requests and the need to provide life-enriching experiences. At ten, the equestrian sport of gymnastics on horseback, Vaulting, took over my life as I became a nationally competitive athlete.

I spent as much time as possible just hanging out at the barn. Leasing a number of horses in my youth gave me the experience of ownership, though ownership didn't materialize until later adulthood. Assisting trainers of dressage and basic English seat, and working in hunter/jumper barns took up much of my time. Working as a "Groom and Administrative and Training Assistant" at a professional hunter/jumper barn in Washington State turned out to be the perfect experience to teach me how to show horses. During that time I rode my Mustang mare on cross-country trails almost every day for the sheer pleasure of it. Years later I bred a sport horse out of her by Ostwind, a champion Hanoverian stallion. The foal hit the ground a perfect mount for me in stature, abilities and temperament. Training his strong spirit and body gave me a deep understanding of the human/equine partnership and helped me develop my training philosophy. I soon preferred working with stallions to mares or geldings. I had to part with him under adverse personal circumstances, but still carry with me the powerful lessons I shared with him.

A part of me stands back, observing all that I do in the human pony play world, and wonders how it happened. My first exposure to human pony play was in 2001 on the Internet while doing research on biological equines; I laughed derisively (it would be an understatement to say that back then my receptivity needed development). Why people would want to play with human ponies when they could have "real" horses was beyond me at the time. I had not yet begun to consider exploring BDSM (bondage and discipline, dominance and submission and sadomasochism). One never knows until one tries. Today I pay off my karma through my deeply entrenched life within the pony play community.

Once BDSM play and kink ignited my life, pony play quickly presented itself again. My first submissive boy gifted me with pony gear purchased from Autumn's

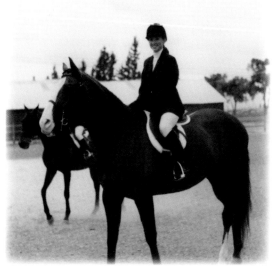

Hunter schooling show, 1992.

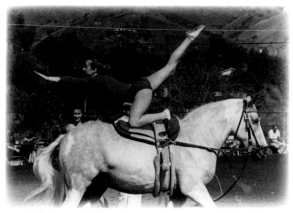

Rebecca and Starr Denison, Horse Vaulting 1983.

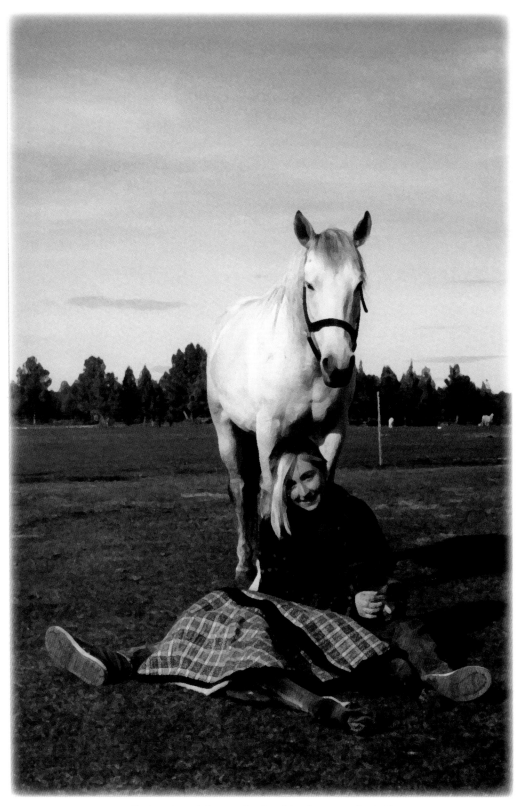

Zack – the mighty stud colt – hits the ground, 1996.

Sub Shop on the Internet because I "like horses so much." I had barely topped him for two weeks when the gift arrived in the mail. So there I was, looking down at him kneeling with his gift in outstretched hands, thinking, "Okay, I have a boy and a human pony harness, and I'm expected to put these things together in a scene somehow." Trying to be a "good" top, I faked confidence and started with trying on the gear to see how it fit. Insecurity about playing kept me from pony play in the beginning. I pushed the gear aside, secretly hoping to enlist help in learning how to do pony play appropriately and according to BDSM tradition. The pony play materials available were scant and turned up little information; I found lots of material about sex, but little else. Intuition demanded more.

After intensely questioning the boy, I found out exactly nothing. The gear made him hot just by looking at it in porn or thinking about having it on, but beyond that it seemed to have little purpose. Wearing the gear alone didn't elicit the same feelings. Apparently the appeal to him had little to do with biological equines. Anne Rice's *Sleeping Beauty* trilogy had set the stage for his pony play fantasies, but, while the fantasies worked well in theory, application seemed out of reach. Tacking the boy up and down with the equipment got boring, as did the miscellaneous bondage scenes with the gear. Serious internet research continued but accomplished little. Even when we joined the local dungeon, Desert Dominion, in Tucson, we found only two ponies, and no trainers.

Eventually I realized if I wanted to play with a pony I had to build the relationship myself from the ground up. I began with what I knew. As an equestrian I knew how to handle a horse, and as a top I knew rudimentary bondage, dominance/submission, and sensory play. My first pony scene commenced where equine knowledge meets sensory play - grooming! Helping to select brushes and such at the local tack shop surprised the boy. As it turned out, he liked grooming a lot! This basic interaction quickly developed into full-fledged training scenes.

Eventually I wanted a cart. Even though possession of a cart seemed a distant possibility, I decided to train with that goal in mind. "Start with the end in mind," Stephen R. Covey's quote from *The 7 Habits of Highly Effective People*, expresses one of the most important concepts of my training philosophy. One must visualize the destination.

The first full pony play scene looked something like this: I captured the pony by throwing a rope around his neck. Using his collar I tied him to the door by running one rope through the crack between the door and his collar, and another rope between the facing door and his collar. That made a makeshift crosstie, with his collar serving as a "halter." The brushes and equipment purchased earlier for sensory play made for perfect grooming. Each brush produced a different sensation. After tacking him up in full pony gear, he learned in-hand work and voice commands. Once the basic commands of "walk-on," "ho," "trot" and "stand" were understood, we moved on to a lunging circle. He learned to extend his gait from the walk to a high step, which looks a little like the conventional BDSM "pony gait" or "parade walk" (some call it "racking"). We moved on to ground driving to prepare to train him to cart.

The session progressed well until he started to get tired and confused. We ended on a good note by reiterating the training process by doing some in-hand work with the voice commands, a strategy that works well in most training conditions. Going back to an easily accomplished level leaves all parties feeling positive about the session once it is over. We ended the training session with cooling down by taking off the tack, but leaving on the headgear without the bit, as you would on a biological equine. Time to relax in my company, during which he received treats and an abbreviated grooming session, rewarded his efforts. My boy had just become my colt-in-training.

The first of many pony play scenes to come, this particular scene flowed elegantly if not without stress. The play tapped into my experience from training and handling biological equines beautifully. It ended up being a good basic scene structure from which I learned a great deal. The demands of the scene proved challenging for a beginning pony; new ponies appreciate a shorter scene. I also came to understand that pony play requires putting aside all preconceived ideas and entering trainer headspace. Luckily for me, I knew that headspace intimately already, and thus had an idea of where to proceed with future sessions.

Over time, this type of play evolved naturally from awkwardness to second nature. Blending my experience with biological equines and BDSM worked. Play with human ponies has become a central play interest for me, and my play style has developed and changed as I have experimented and played with different ponies. I now love sharing my techniques with others. I love all types of ponies and engage in a variety of play dependent upon the pony, my mood, and both of our current interests.

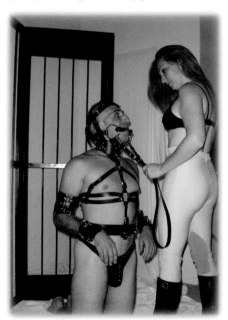

My first pony – ache, 2004.

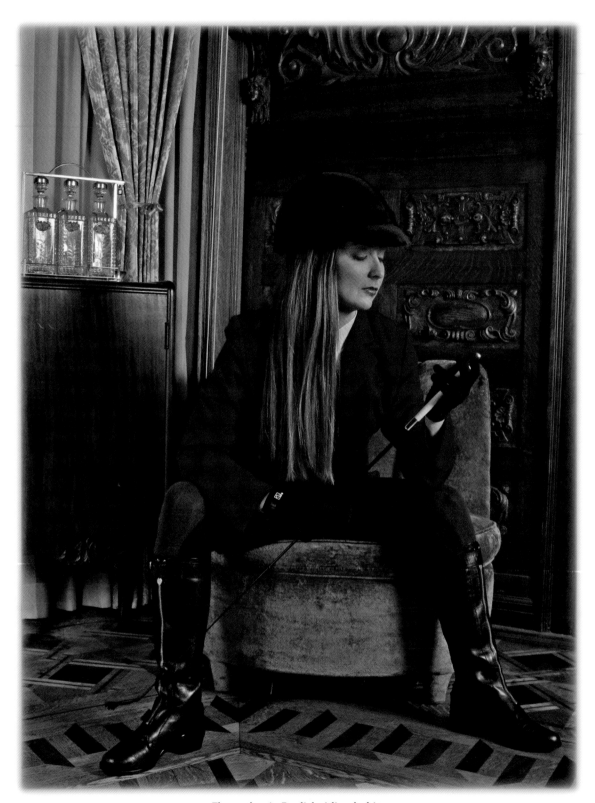

The author in English riding habit.

After the experience in Tucson, I moved to the San Francisco Bay Area for work. Within two weeks I found myself at the Stampede pony munch. There I came to enjoy the fantastic company of other pony players on a regular basis, to share like interests and to plan activities. The ponies and other animal role-players that participate in the munch became invaluable contributors to my development; they opened their lives, gave support, and provided much-needed humor.

As a new transplant to the area, I needed to find like-minded companions. So I volunteered to check out the private property about two hours outside of San Francisco, now known as "The Ranch," for pony play. I quickly became the liaison and de facto leader of pony events at The Ranch in order to get the events off the ground. Thus Ponymistress Rebecca was born.

My pony life now consists of planning events, pony play days, fox hunts and the like; teaching classes; leading discussions; participating on panels; writing; and developing the pony play community in general. Of course, my BDSM interests range far wider than pony play alone, but the uniqueness of pony play speaks to my heart and satiates the deepest passion of my life outside of my family: the love of the horse. Quite unexpectedly, pony play replaced my need for the biological equine. Human pony play feeds my soul in ways nothing else can. With deepest gratitude I thank each pony who has crossed my path for adding to my life in a positive way, especially those who have trusted me to keep them in-hand.

Thank you.

Introduction

The textbook-style presentation of information in this book is designed to facilitate the widest possible range of consensual adult pony play. This book was written to inspire and support a wide span of interests for all players, ponies, trainers, handlers, owners, *et al,* regardless of specifics. It covers the basics of pony play, including helpful exercises to use during self-exploration and negotiations. It explores the "what" and "how" of pony play without dictating right and wrong. It answers questions regarding specific training sessions, how to begin, and basic training philosophy. The philosophy and techniques stand alone, adapting easily to a variety of play.

Training of the biological equine is the key. By emphasizing the information, word choice, and handling and training methods developed by bio-horse trainers over the years, play choices come alive. Some choices work best with certain types of play. For instance, exhibitionists enjoy flashy gear, while someone who prefers to be transformed into a horse may prefer a fuzzy costume that resembles horse hair. The primary philosophy focuses on co-operative gentling methods that use communication, partnership and positive motivation between trainer and pony. Ideally, the relationship guides the play.

Pony role-play provides the opportunity for adults to explore an entirely different side of themselves: a joyful expression of a childlike fantasy game, a wonderfully unique expression of self, entertainment and/or escape. Often it captures a facet of the player's persona that cannot be expressed any other way. Others just like the aspects of fetish or objectification. Sometimes the power exchange of dominance and submission attracts interest. Due to the sheer individuality of expression, no description exhausts the possibilities. Each player finds the type of pony play that speaks to him or her.

Thousands of styles, disciplines, equine types, events and training styles in the biological equine world inspire human ponies.

Because these training techniques for role-play ponies focus on biological equine training, the philosophy adapted to human pony play avoids addressing related elements of play that exceed the primary focus. For example, BDSM, particularly the sadomasochistic (SM) aspect, exceeds that focus. Though many people associate pony play with BDSM, the elements that apply do not define pony play. BDSM easily weaves into pony play for those who wish to use their BDSM talents. Often times BDSM pony play merely puts the bottom in pony gear, but the play engaged in is predominantly BDSM. The distinction made for most animal role-players who also engage in BDSM is whether or not the pony identifies as a pony or as a BDSM role such as a slave, bottom or submissive. In the pony world outside of BDSM, most ponies want to be treated as a biological equine. If the pony identifies as a biological equine, she generally doesn't want to be hit by a whip. (Note: *Equus Eroticus* offers wonderful resources for a lovely combination of SM and role-play ponies.)

The issue of sex also provides a distinction between equine-identified and other players. Many an equine-identified pony regards sex with a human as repugnant or odd; however, a breeding scene with another pony may be exciting. The way that sex fits or doesn't fit into the play challenges the negotiation skills of beginners in the middle of discovering their identification, needs, and wants.

For ease of use, this book includes divisions of information called "Try-Its" and "Training Tips" to highlight training techniques and philosophies. A dictionary of terms, which defines many of the BDSM and equestrian terms used throughout, appears at the back of the book. The appendices provide resources and support material for the player. Other divisions feature important information, such as "Cautions," for emphasis.

The ideas, training philosophy and methods described voice one opinion, based on an equestrian background, to bridge the gap for those without biological equine experience. In this case, a little bit of knowledge encourages perseverance, and the option to take the first step evolves more easily. The ideas presented help to explain the breadth of options available and to encourage the development of a style of play in a fun and individualistic way. Each player only limits their play by the willingness to embrace personal creativity, so *try it*. Keep what feels right and create new things that work. The play truly lends itself to endless creativity. The groundwork and skills illustrated will, I hope, provide ideas for those already engaged in pony play, as well as for novice players who are just getting started.

It's called "play" for good reason – have fun!

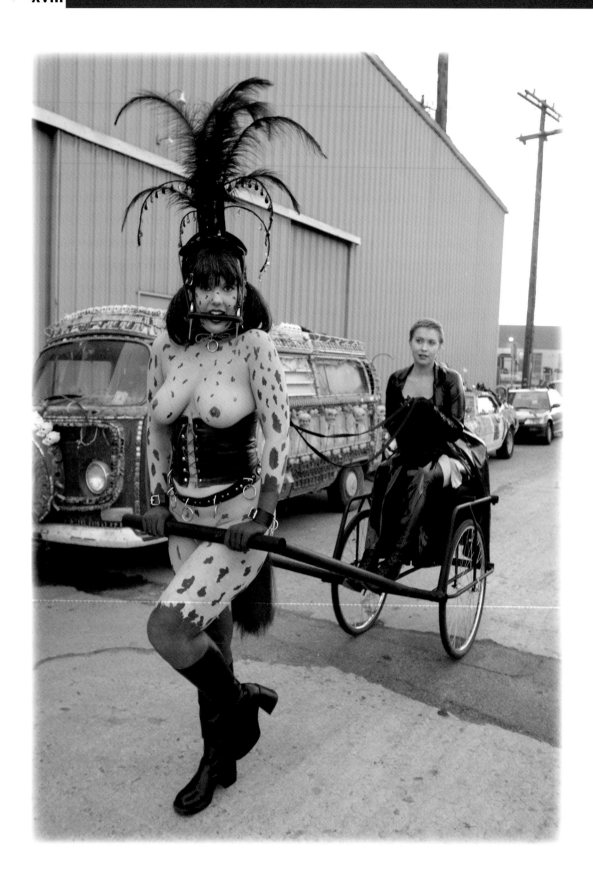

"Pony HeatherLyn and Mistress StarLyn." Photography by Mike Woolson © Woolson www.jumbobrain.com

Chapter One
What Is Pony Play? _____

Pony play defies easy definition. There are as many ways to do pony play as there are ponies, handlers, and the various combinations of each. Some choose to explore pony play as an optional activity aimed at expanding the variety of fun in life. Some choose to express an essential aspect of their persona through becoming a pony. Whenever a human decides to look and act like the biological equine, a form of pony play emerges. The individual defines the motivations and expressions of this type of behavior. Realism and fantasy juxtapose.

Think of the nearly inexhaustible number of breeds and types of biological equines and all the ways they interact with humans: rodeo, farming, war, dressage, three-day eventing, the hunt, pleasure, trail, food, companionship, racing and ranching. Add individual personalities and human interpretation; how could pony play possibly be defined?

However, a few categories of human equines emerge: fetish, SM (sadomasochistic), role-play and furry (sometimes referred to here as equine-identified). Sex may also be used to categorize

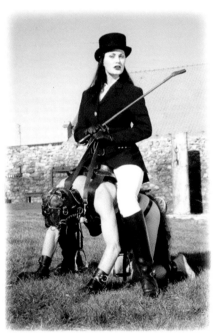

A pony may be on two legs, or a four-legged pony on the ground.

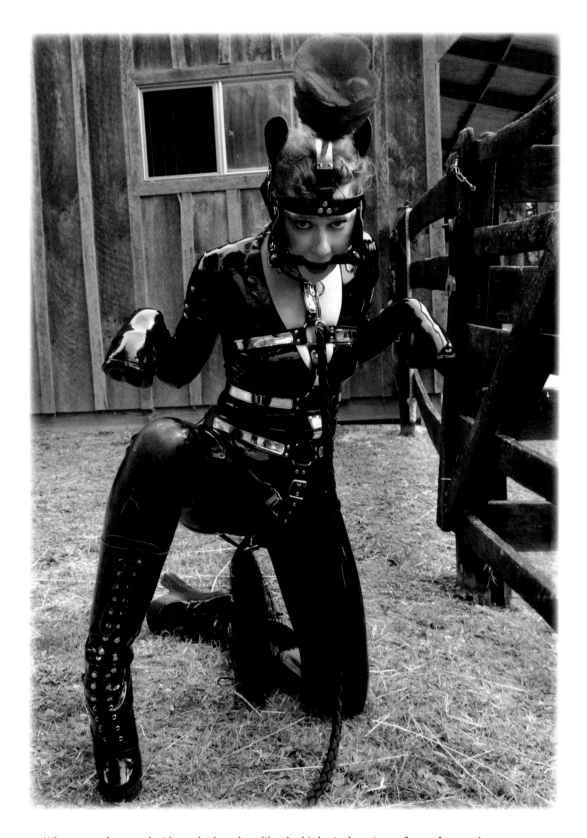

Whenever a human decides to look and act like the biological equine, a form of pony play emerges.

ponies because of its influence on important ethical considerations for play. Some consider sex absolutely integral to the play and others think it distracts from the realism. Ponies occasionally fall into only one category; sometimes they fall into all categories and throw in new interpretations to boot.

Why do people become ponies? Motivations include objectification, exhibitionism, control, denial, sex, play time, emotional vacation, escape, increased imagination, community, relationship, usefulness, service, strength, beauty, and self-expression.

Fetish ponies tend to like the objectification and exhibitionism; a desire for latex encasement is very common. When they cross over with other categories they frequently enjoy being exhibited as role-play show ponies, particularly the ones who are shown in-hand at events. How the "costume" makes them feel, and the perceived responses elicited from the onlookers, often makes the play for them. The type of material and overall look of the costume define the experience. The crowds of people to whom they present themselves reward those who like exhibitionism. Others, in contrast, prefer their privacy and prefer to enjoy their costume alone or with select others.

SM ponies generally express all areas of BDSM: the bondage of the tack, the discipline of the training, the dominance and submission of the handler/trainer-pony relationship and the sadomasochism of the interaction. This is in many ways basic SM, with the added spice of the flattering pony gear or the hot symbolism; people play with it because it gets them off. Sometimes

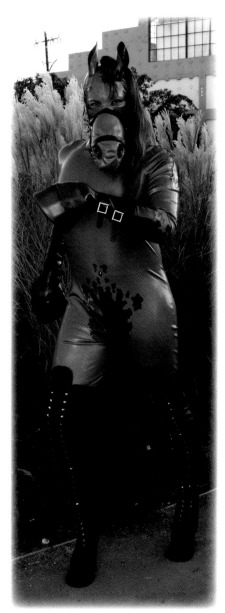

For a "shiny pony" like this, the texture and movement of the attire is part of its pleasure.

Training Tip

Two areas to cover during negotiations:

Q: What kind of pony is this? Is it a sadomasochistic pony interested in sensation, and if so, to what degree? Do bondage, control, and D/S turn the pony on? Does the pony have a specific fantasy to express? To what degree does the pony identify with being an equine? Is it a significant part of the self? What are the characteristics of biological equines that the pony wishes to express?

Q: How does the pony express itself? What does the pony do? What does the play look like in their imagination: show, work, circus, dressage, sport, pet, war, fetish, furry or others? Most importantly, are there any triggers or catalysts that could bring the pony into or out of headspace (that place of reality suspension wherein the human takes on the persona of the horse)?

people choose to play out scenarios about training a resistant pony, requiring whippings and special bondage. Some ponies pride themselves in being "naughty" ponies in order to get worked harder or whipped into obedience; these training sessions build on a forced or pseudo-coercive philosophy of training.

On the other hand, equine-identified ponies do not usually want to be beaten, mishandled or to have sex with humans. The key to determining the appropriateness of SM pony play with a particular pony depends on the type of self-identification the pony has within the context of pony play.

Role-play ponies come in a variety of disciplines: show ponies, draft ponies, cart ponies, work ponies, circus ponies, western ponies, war ponies, companion ponies and more. This type of play comprises one of the largest categories of pony play and encompasses the widest variety of expression; pony role-play frequently crosses over into self-identification with biological equines. Pony players take on being a pony in a way meaningful to them by expressing parts of their personality that may not have other outlets.

Tipsy, a favorite all-around pony of the author, created his own tack and costumery with a flavor all his own, complete with an orange gladiator cingulum, nylon bridle with silver accoutrements, and faux human hair for a tail. Tipsy puts a great deal of energy into his pony persona, including but not limited to his costume, carts, and leading The Stampede pony munch. Role-play ponies generally like to be in a community, or herd. They go to great lengths to put on shows, outings and other events to express the scope of their interests.

Furry ponies generally concern themselves with expressing their identity as horses. The Furry world comprises its own separate community, but in this case the term refers to those identified as equines. The categories within the furry community possess a different context and set of definitions, simplified here for the purpose of this book. Furries choose to express themselves through bringing the animal within to life through behaviors and costumes. Sometimes they express more than one animal, or a fictional creature such as a unicorn or toor. Whereas role-play ponies take on a persona, the furry pony may think of himself as a pony first and a human second. Furry costumes lean toward realism (sometimes cartoon realism, but realism all the same). Usually they want to look as much like a horse or a particular character as possible, often covering the whole body including the head, whereas the SM pony generally likes to be naked under the tack. Examples of fetishists abound in this group as well. For most, bestiality, or zoophilia, does not enter the equation even when having sex amongst other human ponies. Furries comprise a complex and reserved community.

Just as many different kinds of ponies express themselves, handlers/trainers also choose from the same vast possibilities. The interests of trainers parallel similar categories, including dominance and submission (D/S), role-play, partnership, control, bondage, sex and medical play. Some of the various titles include trainer, groom, handler, veterinarian, mistress, master and owner. Their motivations align with the ponies' interests to varying degrees. Each defines his or her identity, knowledge, relationship and type of

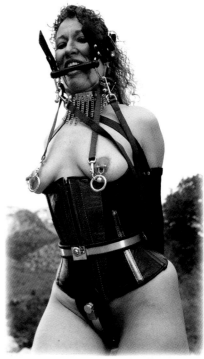

SM ponies do pony play for the symbolism and the sensation.

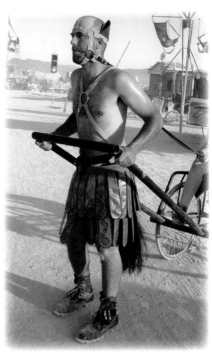

Tipsy shows off his self-created pony tack at the Burning Man Festival.

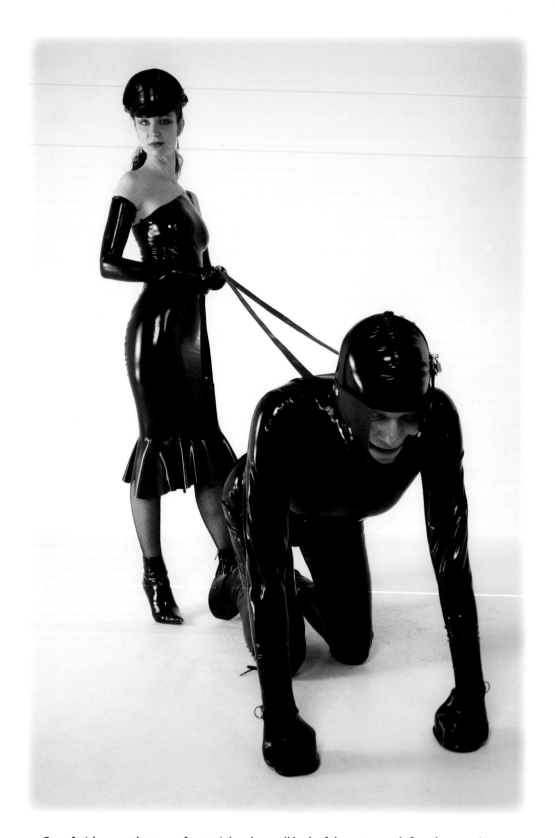

For a fetish pony, the type of material and overall look of the costume define the experience.

Do Your Words Mean The Same Things?

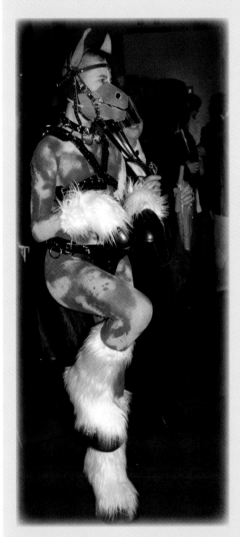

Trainers take the lead in defining the relationship by understanding what the pony needs and wants. They then combine that understanding with what *they* want out of the play, and determine what the play will include. All this must happen through negotiation and explicit consent.

Any of the words we use in pony play can mean different things to different players. Sometimes these differences may drastically impair the final outcome. Take humiliation as a significant and fairly easy example. No activity humiliates universally. Being naked in public horrifies one individual, while another person finds it the most sexually arousing, hottest, and most desired of situations. Some people think of pony play as humiliating, others think of it as the pinnacle of positive self-expression. Defining what words mean to each of the players involved is the first step to effective communication.

If a pony asks a trainer to "train" him, the pony may be asking to be put through his paces with longing and ground driving. However, if the trainer thinks "training" refers to restraining the pony completely between two posts and whipping him, at the very least an upset will result. Neither person will feel satisfied with the play and the pony will likely be confused and dejected. Even more likely, a bewildered trainer may wonder went wrong when the completely irate and violated pony stomps out of the scene without explanation. With careful negotiation, each player's needs can be met, or the decision not to play made proactively before disaster occurs.

One pony experienced confusion with his first experience with pony play. His Mistress decided that training meant verbally degrading and humiliating the pony. He came out of the play feeling like a bad pony. His first try at manifesting his fantasy flopped. If he had collapsed into the feeling that pony play wasn't for him, he wouldn't have continued on to have all the positive experiences he has since had. Luckily, he kept with it and discovered that it just takes the right person or people, as well as thorough negotiation beforehand. Now he plays with people who are interested in the same things and he loves pony play.

Photo: Daisie Dawl and Pony Mistress D.

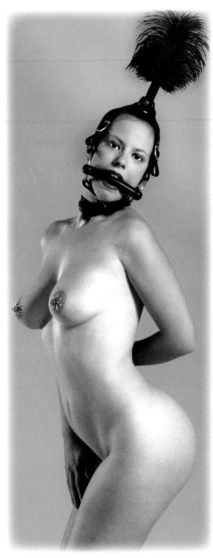

Sexual pony play opens a wide and glorious range of options.

play interests. Some happily own the pony and let others play with it or train it. It's about getting the right match.

As with any other type or play or relationship, negotiating the type of play when ponies and trainers come together plays an important role to the overall success of the scene. It helps to avoid the upset of mismatched expectations, particularly when discussing identity and motivations. Even if interests don't match up, a meeting of minds can occur through careful negotiation.

Sex and sadomasochism exemplify some of the specific, and common, red flags to look out for. Many role-play ponies want to be useful and praised. If a trainer were to get out the whip just for sadistic fun, it may not go over so well with a role-play or an equine-identified pony, and would most likely end the play session in disaster. There seem to be quite a few ponies interested in just being ponies without the sex and sadomasochism. On the other side of the playing field, there seem to be more trainers interested in sex and sadomasochism. Those playing with their sexual partner play in a glorious category with wider options. Each piece influences the negotiations.

First Encounter

When I first met the Pony, he was in a metal shipping crate. A big one – one so large he could live in it. He was on all fours, pacing back and forth, nodding his head in the way that horses do. Occasionally he blew air through his nostrils. He had soft white ears and purple tack that strapped around his jaw and forehead. There was a little silver star just at the top of the forehead. I wanted to touch it. But I was afraid I would spook him. How could I show him that he could trust me?

I had dressed especially for the occasion, as equestrian as I could be in my existing wardrobe. I was wearing a 1940s soft tweed jacket, tailored smartly to my shoulders and waist, tight-fitting black knit pants, and tall black riding boots. In my bag I had packed a few apple slices, in case he was hungry, and something soft to brush him with.

Before this moment, I had only seen the Pony in pictures. One in particular had touched me deeply. In it, he was galloping very fast, so fast that both feet were off the ground and the trees behind him were a blur. He had just a bit of tack on, no pony ears, even, and he was wearing sneakers. But it didn't matter. He was a Pony. You could just see it in his face, and in the gesture of his body. I was surprised by how moved I was. It was something about the effort, the earnestness and the transformation. And something else I hadn't figured out how to name yet.

Now, it wasn't like I had never seen a human Pony before. Years earlier, at the Folsom Street Fair, I spotted my first one, a stunning one. He was dressed head to toe in black shiny leather (or it might have been latex, I wouldn't have noticed the difference, then) except for his chest and thighs, and his entire head was covered in a horsehead mask. His tail bounced up and down as he pranced along. I ran after him, watching him and his proud Owner, exclaiming "Look! A Pony! A Pony!" I was riveted. I felt like a mythological creature had come to life, right there in the street. Something between a minotaur and a centaur: a liminal being. And he was in bondage, and it was really hot.

Another time, as part of a three-evening smorgasbord of spectacular fetish events, I was swimming in all of the hotness surrounding me when I suddenly stopped in my tracks: going by was a whole herd of reindeer girls. They were all linked to one another with rope, lead by a very lean and handsome Santa. And, yes, they were deer and not ponies, but they looked remarkably equine, dressed in little more than a few white fur tufts here and there, flanks gleaming, breasts jingling, forelegs raised just like hooves. One of them coyly wiggled her hindquarters and winked at me, and I thought I might faint. I really didn't know if I wanted to be her or have her, but at the time just watching was stimulation enough.

But this Pony was different. I saw it in the pictures. He was just a horse, ready to do horse things. I couldn't imagine smacking him or whipping him or putting him in black

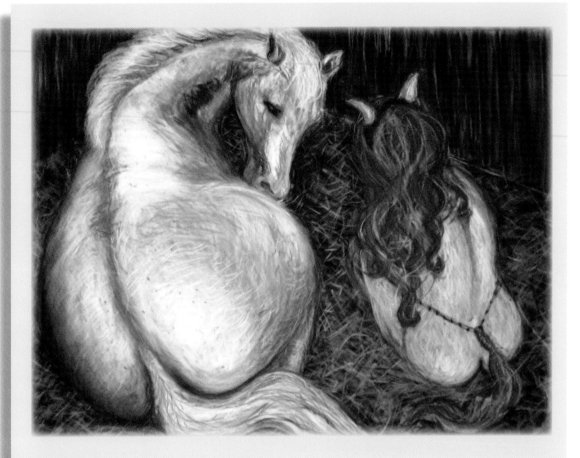

leather bondage, which was something I had always associated with human ponies before that. And since I am the sort of gal who takes as much pleasure as the next kinky person in such things, I was surprised that this wasn't coming up for me with him. If anything, I felt extremely protective. I wanted to keep him safe.

Back in the crate, the Pony continued to pace. He kept his head down, but I knew he was aware of me. He seemed curious and a little afraid at the same time. He was so big – a horse – but also so exposed. I was suddenly very shy. Everything was so quiet. I put out my hand and called his name. I told him what a pretty pony he was. He pressed his muzzle into my palm. I felt the strength of him, and the gentleness. A little shiver went up my spine. I could feel something start to melt in me, and in him.

I scratched him behind the ears, his sweet white ears, and he pressed into me harder, nearly knocking me over, the way big dogs do. I laughed and sat down. I offered him my slices of apple which he slurped up out of my hands. It tickled and I laughed some more. I began talking to him like I was a little girl and he was my first animal friend. I gave him a big bowl of water that he pushed his big head in and drank out of, then pulled back and shook himself off, splashing droplets all over himself and me.

"The Visitor," Illustration by Daisy Eneix – © 2006

I remember, when I was little, walking in the woods, trying to catch wild things. You had to be quiet and wait, and listen. You had to be gentle. It's like what they say about Unicorns. That if you want to meet one you have to sit and wait under a tree, quiet, and somehow be gentle and still enough that he will risk coming out from his hiding place, and come to you, and put his head in your lap.

The Pony put his head in my lap. I had a soft glove that I rubbed against him, and he liked that. There was a grooming brush nearby, and I started brushing him. I started with his tail, but it looked fragile, so I moved on to his back, his hindquarters and his legs. He stretched his body so that I could reach different parts of him more easily. He seemed half-wild, half-tame, like an abandoned farm horse. I could tell he had missed the human contact.

He started to get restless. He got up and walked and pranced around a bit, even jumping a little. I wanted to try riding him, but wasn't sure if he was ready for that. When he started nosing at my legs, I thought that was a sign, and I straddled his back. He did not try to throw me, but lifted me easily.

When I was about eleven years old, I dreamed that I climbed up onto a Pegasus and flew around the world. I held onto him as he leaped up higher and higher, and when I peeked over his shoulder I could see the oceans and the mountains and the clouds below me. Normally I was afraid of heights, but on this creature's back I felt totally safe. I knew I wasn't going to fall. This was the closest thing I had to a flying dream.

Riding this Pony was a little awkward at first. I didn't want to hurt his back, so I sat closer to his rump, with my legs dangling on either side of him. But I felt unwieldy and he knew it. He started pawing at my boots with his front hooves, and I realized that, unlike non-human horses, I could actually wrap my legs all the way around him. I crossed my boots underneath him, the leather pressing against his flanks and my thighs clinging to his back. He walked a circle and I held onto his back also with my hands, feeling the sensation and trying not to tip.

At one point he stood still and began to shift, forward and back, in place. I couldn't tell what he was doing. I wanted not to fall, but I found myself sliding, back and forth, up and down his back. Where was he going with this? My endorphins figured it out before I did, sending up waves of pleasure from between my legs all the way up my spine, until I came, all over his back, slick and wet and trembling. Oh. Smart pony. Good Pony.

Before that, I hadn't really known if it was all right to do sexual things with a human Pony, especially one that seemed so real. Well, it was. At least with this one. And so, we spent the rest of the afternoon exploring, with him being a very friendly Pony, and me being a very curious little Girl.

And that was how I first met my Pony. It was a big beginning.

– Juliana Switch

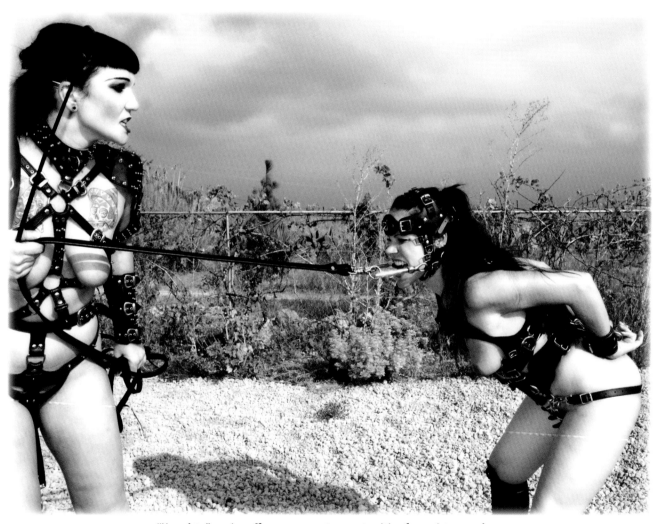

"Naughty" ponies offer some great opportunities for resistance play.

Chapter Two
Pony and Trainer Headspace

Players often talk about headspace. The umbrella term "headspace" refers to a variety of mental and emotional conditions that the player identifies as the particular frame of reference from which he or she operates while playing. There are several levels of headspace, each correlating with a certain degree of disengagement from an everyday frame of reference or with the intensity of the experience.

Entering fantasy role-play suspends one's social identity and everyday persona. The experience can range from superficial make-believe to complete suspension of everyday reality such that there is no memory of hearing human language or making human meaning out of the events taking place. "Headspace" generally implies a particularly intense level of concentration. Most players desire a deeper sense of headspace when playing, as play brings the mind to a deeper level of connection and greater suspension of human reality.

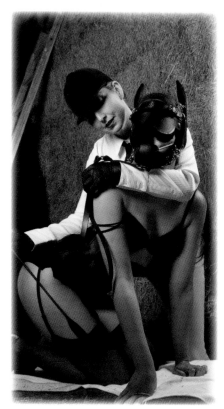

Play brings the mind to a deeper level of connection and greater suspension of human reality.

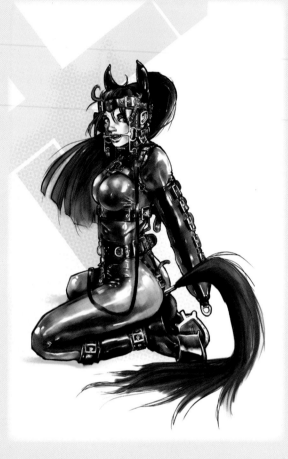

Ponygrrl

My first exposure to pony play occurred when I ran across a story about a pony girl while reading erotic literature on the Internet. In the story women were transformed into ponies through restrictive attire and domination. They became subhuman sex-slaves. I read several stories afterward. They aroused me intensely and became one of my favorite fantasies, since BDSM and humiliation are among my primary fetishes.

Imagine my surprise when I learned a few years later that pony play is not limited to the fantasy scenarios of erotica. Learning about people who willingly act as ponies as a form of expression in real time intrigued me. It surprised me even more to find out it doesn't necessarily involve sex or eroticism. I never realized pony play was so broad.

I have to admit that, even as my knowledge of this role-play expands, I am still most interested in the BDSM aspect. Perhaps a weak self-identity and lack of imagination hold me back from expressing myself as a pony merely for the sake of expression. As interesting as the range of pony play is, I would likely be most interested in being a submissive, sex-slave pony when I finally decide to engage in pony play.

– M.H.

"Ponygrrl" illustration by Punchyninja

Some ponies enter headspace merely by being called by their pony name and scratched behind the ear. Others need gear to trigger the response. Adding costuming, such as ears and a tail, can be powerful headspace triggers. For those with tack, taking the bit can be a powerful trigger as well. Occasionally an entire ritual of preparation must take place for full effect. It takes a little trial and error for the green pony to find the right activities to get into an appropriate frame of mind. Handlers and trainers must also go through a similar process of discovering what works for them.

Both ponies and trainers engage their minds in a conditioning of behaviors associated with the character, or role, they take on. A self-identified pony continues to develop that persona, just as a human evolves through everyday experiences.

Desire goes only so far. It takes research to gain the knowledge necessary to play within the realm of equestrian disciplines. Eventually a cycle of application and evaluation takes the play to a deeper level.

So what does it take to be a trainer? Beyond possessing a willing pony, basic gear, and the basic scene organization for a training session, it takes gumption. "Gumption," according to Webster, is a bold shrewdness in practical matters that includes common sense and courage, and is useful in initiating an enterprise. The biological equine world calls it "horse sense." Equestrians tend to posses a no-nonsense, practical way about them that gets things done. Put it together for a formula for fun.

A trainer decides either to develop and persevere with a particular interest and training style, or to adapt his or her personal style to various ponies. It helps if the trainer asks the same questions of herself that she asks of the pony. When the trainer understands her

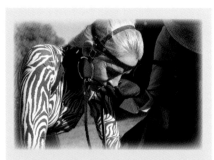

Try-It: Developing Headspace

Reflect on what pony play looks like to you. What image or feeling comes to mind when you think of pony play? Maybe it's a sound or smell. How does the fantasy make you feel? Shut your eyes for a minute to get a clear sense of the key elements to you. What are the roles and experiences implied in that sensual experience? Do you see a specific breed of pony running through the woods tossing her mane in the breeze? Can you feel the harness on your body or the gear in your hands? Do you smell the leather, latex, or carrots? Can you hear someone telling you what a good pony you are? Do you command, or cue, the pony to do a trick? Are you strutting your stuff in front of a crowd or are you in a quiet barn at night? Clarify the vision by writing it down for ease of communication to someone else, perhaps a potential play partner.

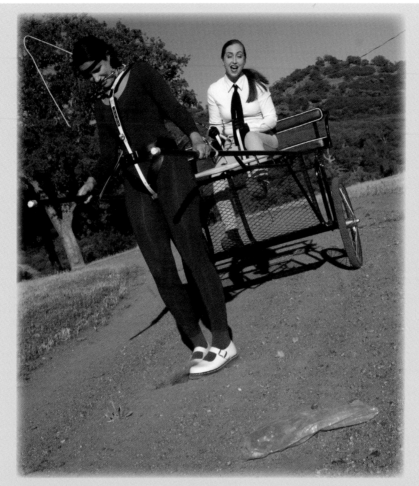

Training Tip

Think like a pony: When your friend, lover, play partner, submissive, masochist, or slave enters pony head space, he or she has literally become the pony, along with everything ponyhood means to them. The expression of that persona produces new and often unexpected behaviors, sometimes altogether different from everyday behavior. For example, your otherwise very sensible, self-reliant girlfriend may jump and shy away from a startling noise when she's a pony. She may even run off (now the round-up begins!).

Deep headspace may render the pony unable to respond from a rational, human mindset, and may leave her unable to take care of herself. In fact, most ponies suspend verbal communication and adopt a nonverbal communication system. The runaway pony in the example above would be non-verbally communicating her fear, choosing to flee danger precisely as a prey animal would.

This means that as a trainer or handler, you must listen with your ears, your eyes and your intuition. As the trainer, the responsibility lies with you to think ahead and create a safe space for your pony. As your bond with the pony develops, the pony will learn to trust you. When that occurs, you become the source of protection and the pony learns it is safe to stay with you instead of running off. Just watch your feet; they may get stepped on when she runs to you for protection!

Try-It - Pony Homework

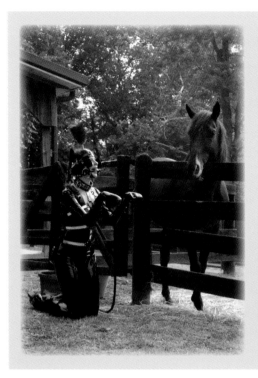

Design or acquire costuming that best expresses your personality and inner desires. Research and decide on a specific breed. It does matter. Breeds illuminate and expand personality traits and sometimes the function of expression.

Observe biological equines. Human ponies gain a tremendous amount of knowledge by observing biological equines to get a feel for how they interact with each other and with humans.

Read horse stories, look at equine-inspired art, or find other modalities that speak to you. Inspiring folklore as well as popular culture horse stories add to the understanding of biological equines and their world.

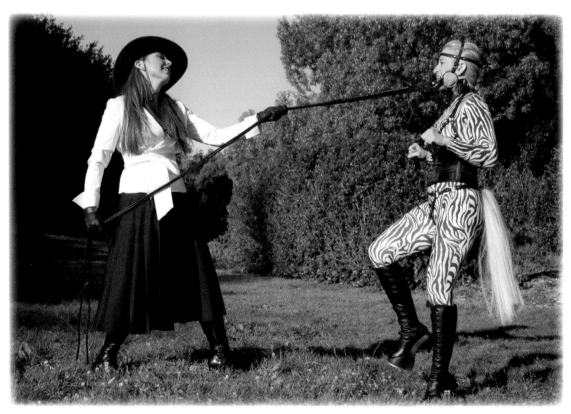

Serious resistance, or playful tug-of-war? It all depends on the headspace of pony and trainer.

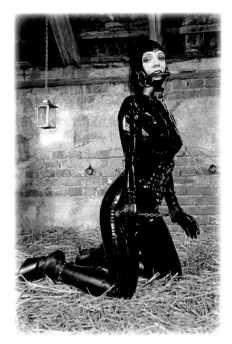

Entering fantasy role-play suspends one's social identity and everyday persona.

interests and motivations, she has a better understanding about what kind of pony she would enjoy playing with. The trainer must know what she wants to get out of the play to be able to create the environment and elicit the behavior.

Training a pony takes dedication to research. The best trainers explore their own desires and fantasies as deeply as their ponies do, reading how-to books, training manuals, magazines, and websites by trainers from the biological equine world. Both good information and conflicting information exist side by side; these represent options for creating an individual style that works for trainer and pony. One trainer's methods might speak to a given individual more clearly than another's. The endless variety of options in the biological equine world parallels the options in the human pony play world. Explore, try it, and keep what resonates.

Chapter Three
Equipment

Equipment includes everything necessary to engage in the desired pony activities.

Human pony players usually include their "costume" in the equipment list. Costumes may include all or none of the following: ears; tail; skin suit of furry material, latex, spandex or other textile; clothing or lack thereof; and hooves.

Tack enables the pony to be put to use. Basic tack includes bit, bridle, saddle, harness, and reins. Any biological equine tack can be adapted or used as a design for human pony tack.

Training aids, such as spurs, whips, martingales and the like, provide ways to keep the pony's attention. Using a whip, for example, creates a learning situation that later in training becomes a physical, auditory, and visual aid.

Other necessary equipment depends upon the discipline. A Western Quarter Horse pony might need barrels for barrel racing, poles for pole bending, and little critters (biological or human) to round up. Dressage ponies need a dressage arena,

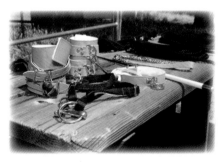

Equipment need not be ornate or expensive. A few basic items available at any good erotic boutique may be enough to get you started.

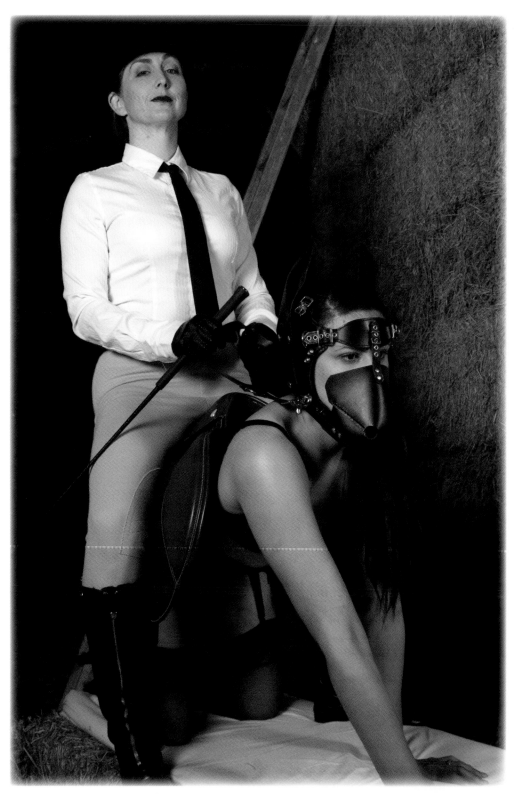

A well-equipped pony and trainer are a happy and proud pony and trainer.

and Jumpers need obstacles. Rodeo broncos need an eight-second clock to time the competition.

The gear contributes to positive head-space, training resources and general allure. Requirements for individual ponies vary according to the pony's personality, interests, discipline and functions. Internet sources provide a wide variety of equipment and tack, covering everything from custom designed and fitted gear to common factory gear. It's possible to put together a full costume in a couple of hours on the internet to with the price tag in the $600-$5,000 range. Alternatively, many players design and make their own pony gear and equipment – with a little creativity, something can be put together in a couple of weekends for $50-$200. The overall objective guides the final decision.

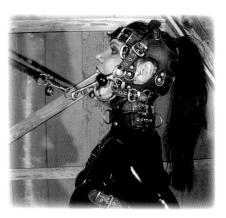

Requirements vary according to the pony's personality and functions.

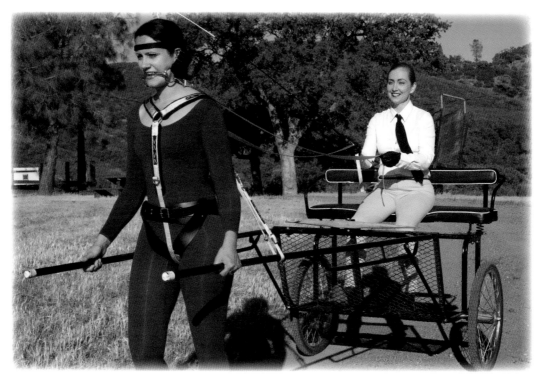

Equipment made for biological equines can easily be adapted for their human counterparts. All the equipment in this photo is from a tack shop.

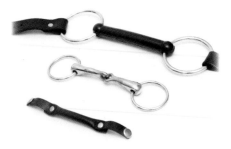

Bits vary widely in size and style.

Most pony gear functions as bondage, whether it's intended for BDSM play or not. All bondage must be treated as such, with all safety considerations taken into account. For those unfamiliar with bondage safety procedures, please research bondage techniques carefully, and only utilize techniques within your individual comfort and competency. Some bondage teaching resources are listed in the Resource Guide.

Human ponies customarily develop a costume that expresses their pony persona. While some ponies require nothing to enter headspace and play, others require a complex ritual, including covering their bodies from head to toe in costume, whether that be leather, spandex, latex, fur or otherwise. Body painting provides another option. More fanciful ponies may sport wings, unicorn horns, ribbons, or bells. Three basic equipment essentials for virtually all ponies are ears, a bit, and a tail.

Basic Training Aid Kit

Bit – controls head and communicates cues

Lead line – In-hand control

Reins – directional communication for dressage, reining, cart, and various disciplines

Whips – communicate space, body awareness, emphasizes directives and commands, and give a general cue for movement, as most ponies will move away from contact with the whip

Restraints (bondage) – for headspace, body control, appearance, discipline…

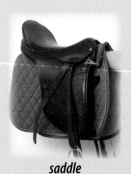

saddle

Martingale – holds head in place

Side reins – holds head in place

Saddle – provides comfortable platform for riding

Spurs – emphasize cues

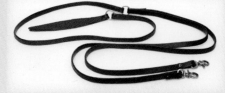

reins

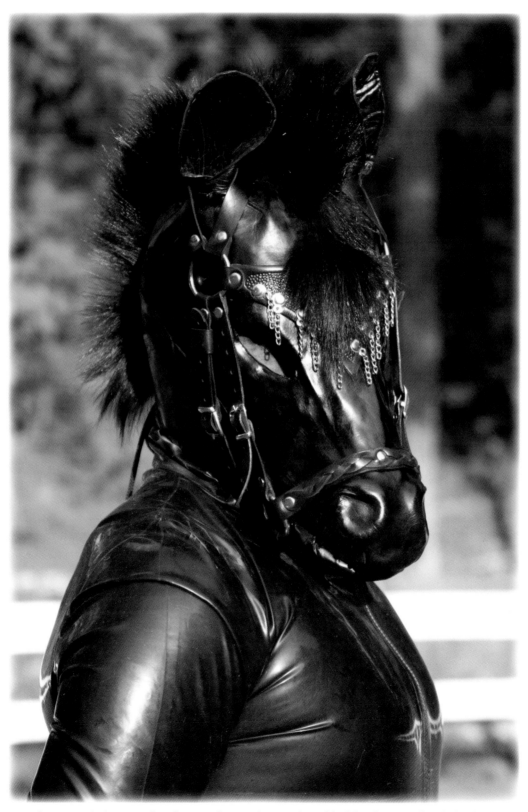

Just try resisting pony headspace when you're wearing a black leather pony hood like this!

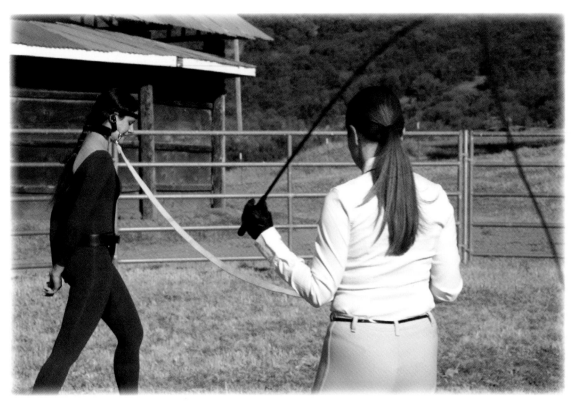

Working on the lunge line is
wonderful for warmup and practice.

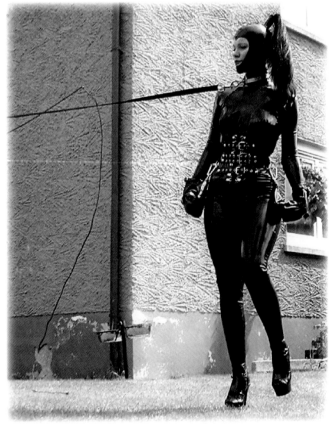

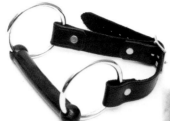

A bit may be made for human mouths, like one of these (left and below)...

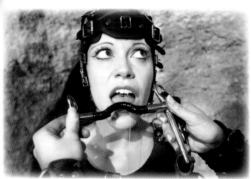

... or you can adapt an equine snaffle for human use by using a special wrap (far right) or wrapping it in a sport bandage (below) to protect your pony's teeth.

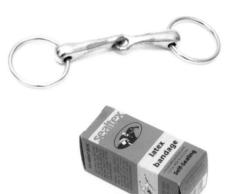

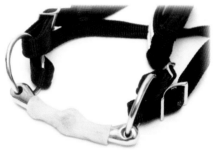

On the left is a full biological equine nylon bridle which has been adapted to the human pony, whereas the ProDeviant bridle on the right was made especially for human use.

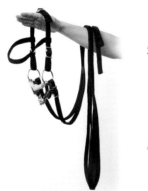

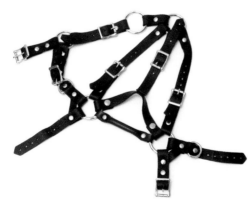

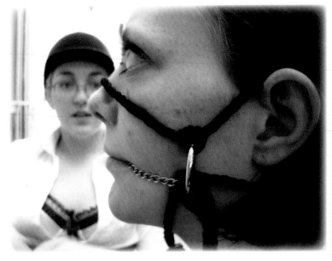

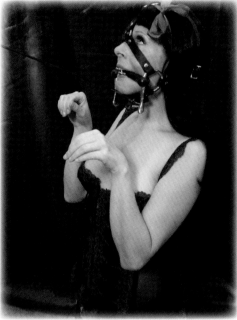

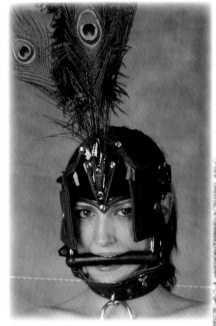

A good bridle may be
homemade from a few lengths of
cord and chain, or an elaborate
custom creation costing many
hundreds of dollars.

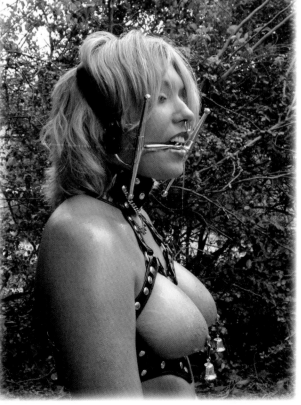

Clockwise from top: Custom rope bridle made by a friend of Strawberry pony, photographer Joni Gear. "Autumn in comfort-fit rubber bit gag and training harness-headstall," www.sub-shop.com, © 2007 sub-shop.com. Biological equine full cheek snaffle bit, photo by Shadowplayers.com, © 2007 Shadowplayers.com. Headstall variation, photo by Shadowplayers.com, © 2007 Shadowplayers.com.

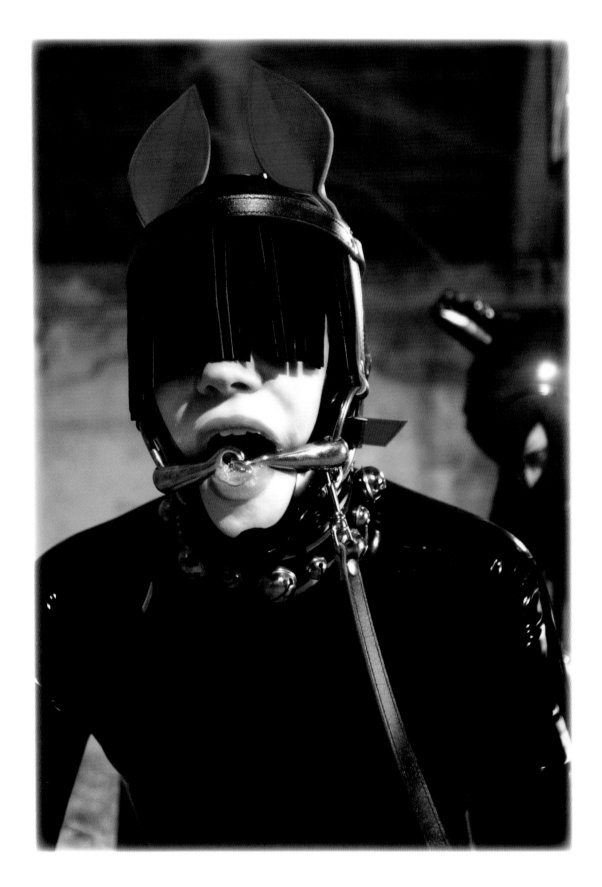

Pupett in equine snaffle bit, © Matthias Kohl; Pupett is a registered trademark of Matthias Kohl.

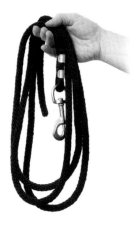 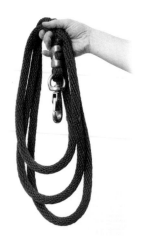 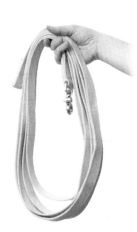

Left: a llama lead rope, very comfortable for human ponies. Center: a heavy-duty equine lead rope which would be more challenging. Near left: a bio-equine lunge line modified for the shorter distances of human pony play.

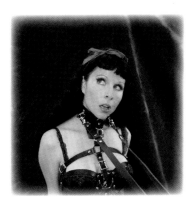 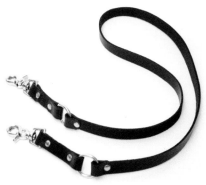

Right: short human pony reins. Above: reins attached at collar for leading.

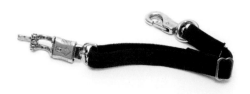 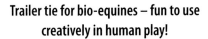

Trailer tie for bio-equines – fun to use creatively in human play!

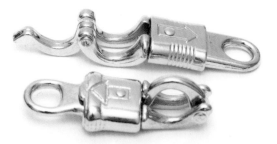

Panic snaps are an important addition to your safety gear, facilitating quick release of tie-downs.

Tack primarily suits ponies in training. Though the pony may like it for looks, tack functions as training equipment.

The most popular tack item represented is the bit. Bits appeal to most human ponies and trainers, as they provide the key to communication, connection and control.

To use a bit, you need reins. Harnessing falls in line next in order of popularity. Equipment used to control, communicate with, or to make the pony useful reinforces the function of the pony itself and the relationship with the handler or trainer. The trainer and equipment matches the chosen discipline regardless of who does the choosing.

Cart ponies need a cart. A harness, driving reins, and cart whip add to the fun. Trick ponies need obstacles, perhaps orange cone patterns and agility tests. Work ponies, sometimes known as draft ponies, need loads to haul and possibly special harnesses.

Gearing up applies to handlers and trainers as well. Handlers and trainers possess attire and equipment designating their interests and disciplines. A hunt mistress might don the traditional Pinque coat, white breeches, black boots and cap. Rodeo riders generally prefer cowboy hats, jeans, chaps and western boots. Veterinarians provide a medical setup as part of their play. Grooms require specialized equipment. Handlers sometimes choose to have a special outfit, especially when showing the pony.

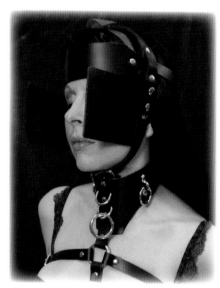

Blinders screen out distractions without impeding vision.

Windy

I have been interested in pony play for most of my kinky life. One day I read about an outing by the group that was later to become Stampede, so I grabbed my human pet and off we went. Once there, we got dressed up; then I handed her the reins and said, "Now you are my handler." She is a good girl and willing to do my bidding, so after a quick explanation she remembered how she handled bio-horses when she was younger. That and the rest of the very helpful folk at the event made for a very pleasant afternoon.

My original interest in pony play was mainly in the heavy bondage restraint you see in pictrures of pony girls, often tied to stable walls or to a walker or cart. However, I have since come to appreciate two other elements: the care and protectiveness of the handlers and trainers, and the uniqueness of pony headspace. I cannot describe it in English and you likely can't speak the language of horses. English does not even have a word that means horse language.

In 2000, The Stampede hosted a dog and pony show at Castlebar in San Francisco. I was entered in the show by my trainer Emerald. It was at that show that I developed my costume from its early stages to my now characteristic reddish body suit, homemade and store-bought bondage elements, and pony girl headpiece. I also found the first taste of pony headspace. I am a very shy person and going out to perform in front of the crowd was at first very hard. I also hate to lose. To combat these human emotions I concentrated on being a horse. I realized that as a pony, I was interested only in pleasing my trainer and didn't t care at all about the show as long as I got fed and groomed.

Today, my trainer Rebecca and I share a strong human/pony bond forged of her skills as a trainer of bio horses and my constantly evolving abilities to let go of my ego and human concerns and "just be."

– Windy

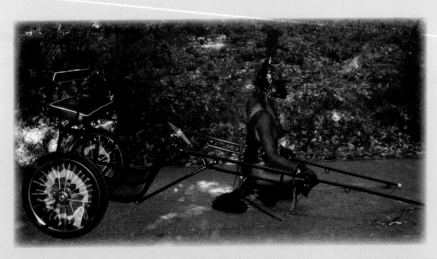

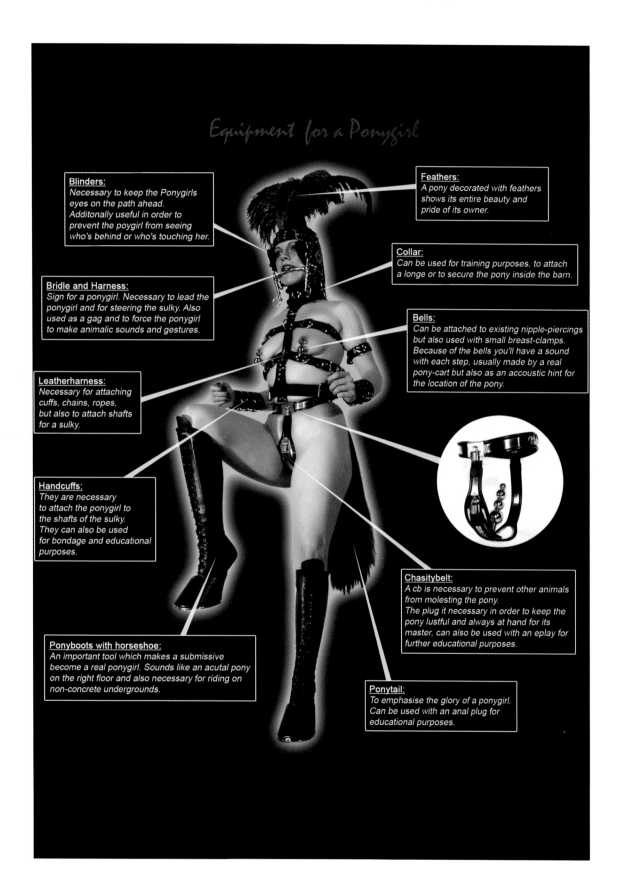

Equipment for a Ponygirl

Blinders:
Necessary to keep the Ponygirls eyes on the path ahead. Additonally useful in order to prevent the poygirl from seeing who's behind or who's touching her.

Bridle and Harness:
Sign for a ponygirl. Necessary to lead the ponygirl and for steering the sulky. Also used as a gag and to force the ponygirl to make animalic sounds and gestures.

Leatherharness:
Necessary for attaching cuffs, chains, ropes, but also to attach shafts for a sulky.

Handcuffs:
They are necessary to attach the ponygirl to the shafts of the sulky. They can also be used for bondage and educational purposes.

Ponyboots with horseshoe:
An important tool which makes a submissive become a real ponygirl. Sounds like an acutal pony on the right floor and also necessary for riding on non-concrete undergrounds.

Feathers:
A pony decorated with feathers shows its entire beauty and pride of its owner.

Collar:
Can be used for training purposes, to attach a longe or to secure the pony inside the barn.

Bells:
Can be attached to existing nipple-piercings but also used with small breast-clamps. Because of the bells you'll have a sound with each step, usually made by a real pony-cart but also as an accoustic hint for the location of the pony.

Chasitybelt:
A cb is necessary to prevent other animals from molesting the pony. The plug it necessary in order to keep the pony lustful and always at hand for its master, can also be used with an eplay for further educational purposes.

Ponytail:
To emphasise the glory of a ponygirl. Can be used with an anal plug for educational purposes.

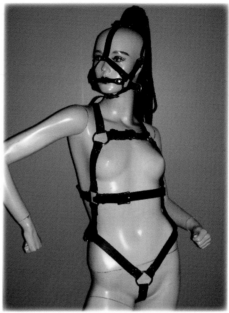

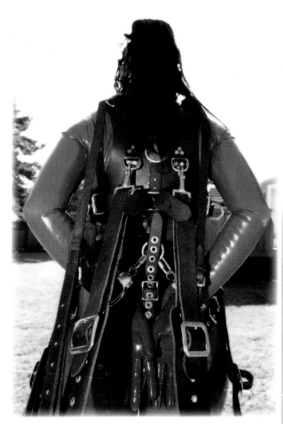

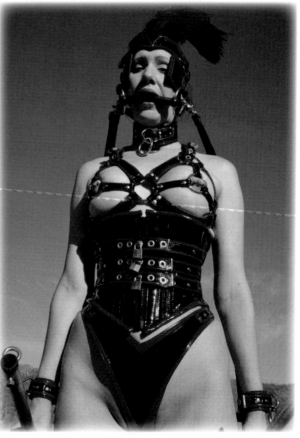

Clockwise from left, this page: Plow harness photo © Matthias Kohl, Pupett is a registered trademark of Matthias Kohl. On mannequin, ProDeviant.com pony tack – deluxe pony headstall and body harness. Photos courtesy of ProDeviant.com, © ProDeviant.com, all rights reserved. Corset and Harness, photo by Shadowplayers.com, © 2007 Shadowplayers.com.

Practical or fetishistic? Adjustable for many ponies or custom made for one? Choose the harness that fits the needs of both trainer and pony.

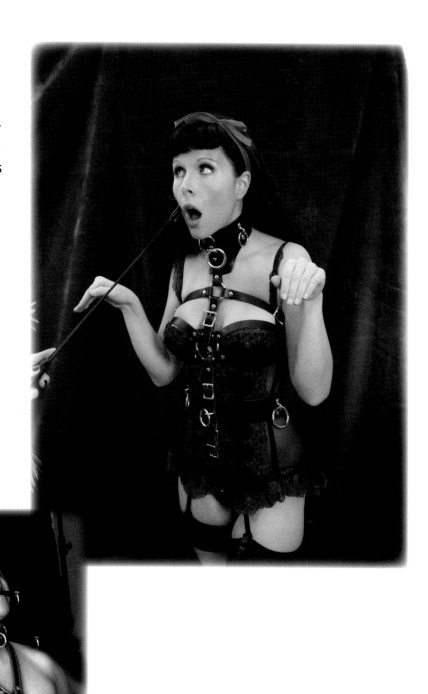

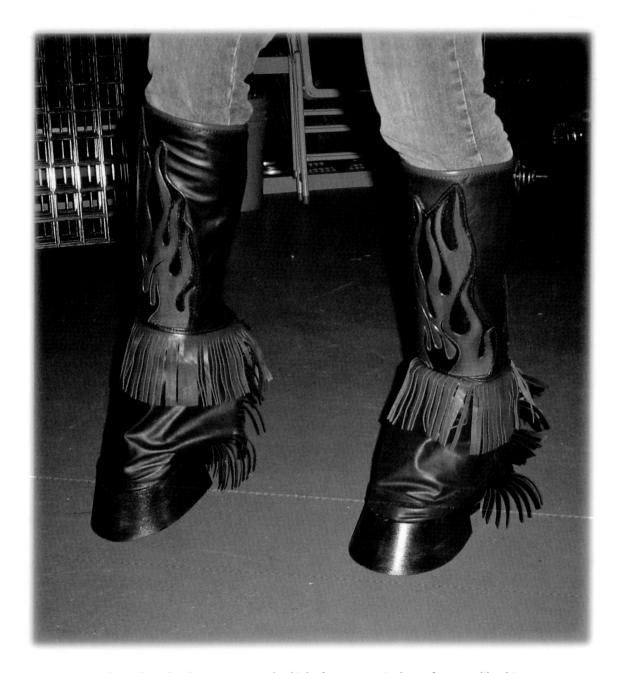

When a boot fetish meets a pony play kink, the outcome is showy footwear like this.

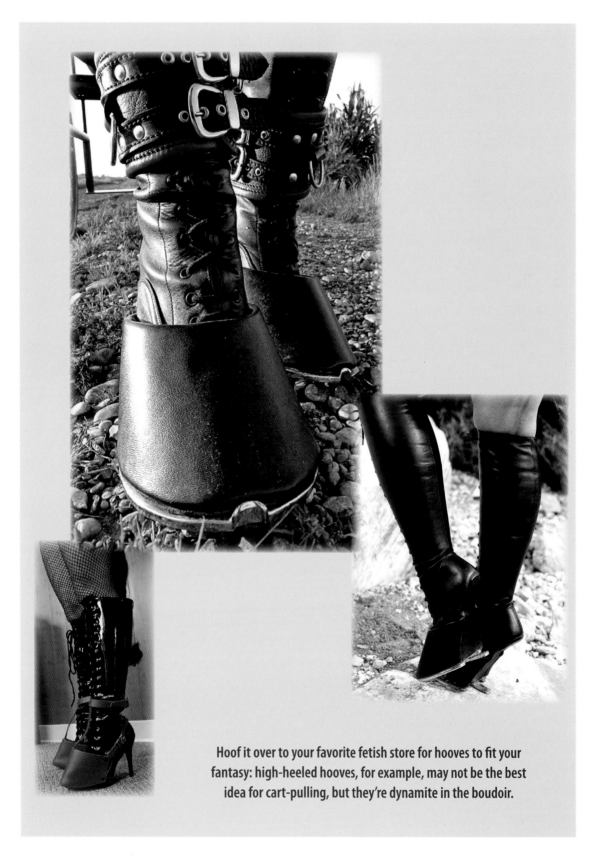

Hoof it over to your favorite fetish store for hooves to fit your fantasy: high-heeled hooves, for example, may not be the best idea for cart-pulling, but they're dynamite in the boudoir.

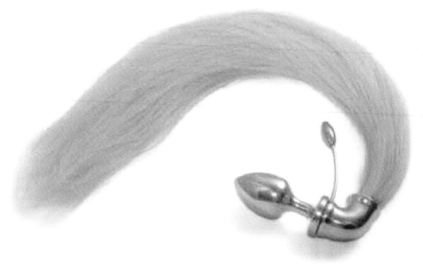

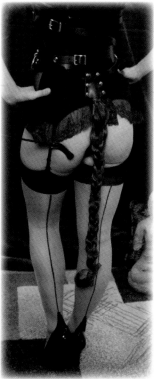

Tails may be strap-on or insertable, and made from horsehair, human hair, artificial hair or anything else that fits your fantasy.

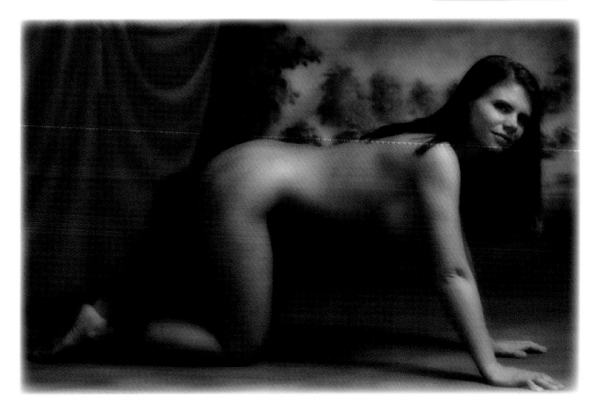

Top: Plug, courtesy of Rupert Huse & Son, Inc., www.huse.com. Harness tail by www.Sub-shop.com, © 2007 Sub-Shop.com. Bottom: Model on all fours, courtesy of Rupert Huse & Son, Inc., www.huse.com.

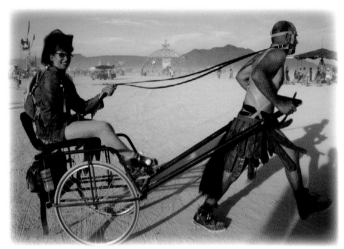

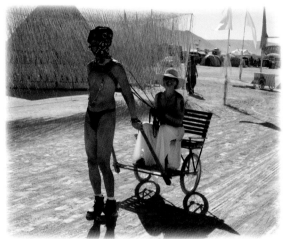

Cart styles may vary depending on
the strength and number of ponies
and the style of the scene.

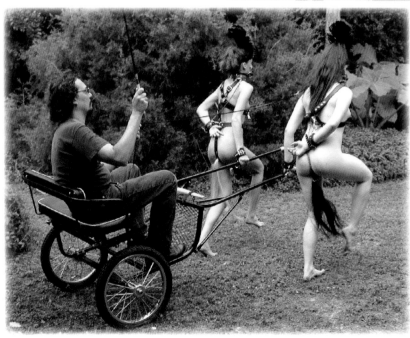

From top: Photo by Mike Woolson, © 2007 Woolson, www.jumbobrain.coom.
Pony and mistress at Burning Man. Photographer unknown.
Photo courtesy www.Shadowplayers.com, © 2007 Shadowplayers.com

I've been interested in pony play since I was pretty young. At that time there was nothing sexual about it – I was just a girl pretending to be a pony. My best friend was a Thoroughbred mare named Peaches, and I've been around and on horses since I was a toddler, so naturally, I would emulate them in as many ways as I could get away with.

As a child, I showed equines through 4-H, FFA, open shows and breed circuits in everything from on the ground to jumping and dressage. I also drove the ponies, so I'd often pull my brother and friends around the barn in the sulky. I've even had the pleasure of raising foals from birth through their riding years.

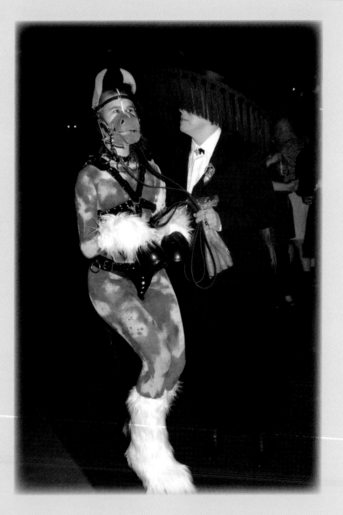

As I grew up, I would use the equine spirits to help me out. To push my body into training to be faster, I often imagined I was a wild mustang; soon, with that thought, I became one of the fastest kids in my junior high school. I also pranced around on beaches to raise my spirits.

Thinking like a work horse helps work go by faster. But I mainly do it to be closer to the equine species. I moved from horse country to the city, and I felt so separated from horses, I feel it helped me to keep sane in this crazy fast-paced world.

I do pony play because I love and respect equines. I put a skin on and design my horse persona to help me feel more like a horse, as well as to help others view me more as a horse. I could go off on a long tangent about horses and why they are such incredible animals, but I think it's humble to stop here.

– Daizie Dawl

Photo: Daizie Dawl and Pony Mistress D.

Chapter Four
Training Your Pony _____

Trainers need to determine their training style and expectations early on in the trainer-pony relationship. Creating the perfect pony requires a clear vision of the perfect pony, including desired behaviors.

Just as humans need to consider socio-cultural elements when communicating with each other, pony players have to think about their own values when it comes to developing the relationship between pony and handler. What behavior does the trainer consider okay for a pony to have?

On the other side of the equation, the pony must consider the range of behaviors and level of performance the handler desires, and the quality of manners the trainer hopes to instill. Obviously the owner/partner and pony relationship involves more intimacy and casual interaction than two players who have just met. A more casual relationship may focus more on training than personal interaction. The relationship dynamic of various ponies and handlers depend upon the interests and relationship involved; there is no "right" dynamic.

Every pony, whether human or biological, possesses a unique personality. The biological equine

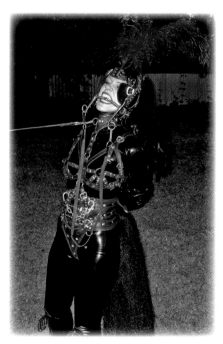

Every pony, human or equine, possesses its own personality.

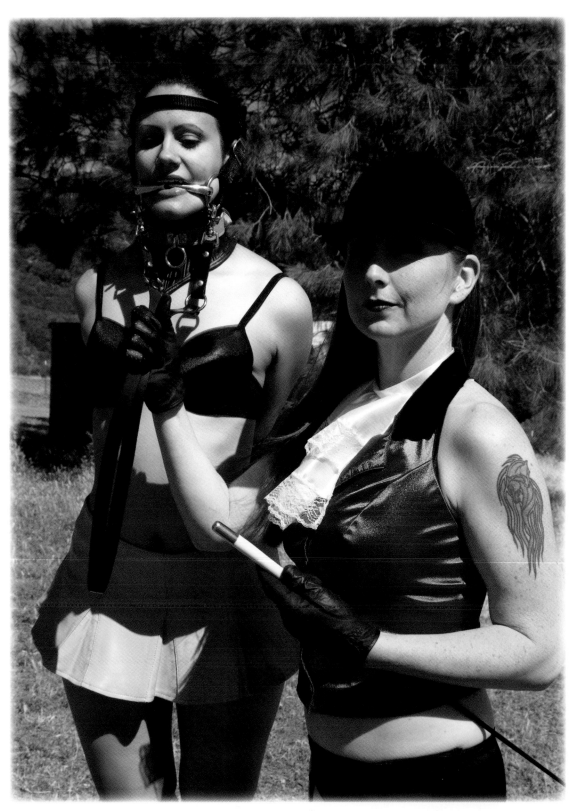

A well-trained pony is a joy and a souce of pride for both the trainer and the pony itself.

does not possess self-awareness, only a will and instinct: a green-broke biological equine appears lost sometimes because it does not understand what's going on. The human, on the other hand, consciously projects himself into his pony persona and/or creates a persona. Some ponies retain a single pony identity; others may carefully research and create several personas. Sometimes personalities evolve over time; this evolutin can take place during play, without conscious control.

The trainer can manage how the pony interacts with others, referred to as community behavior; how it interacts with its handler or trainer, or in-hand behavior; and how it responds to learning specific behaviors, or training to a discipline.

Community behavior. The pony's character emerges through its actions within the community

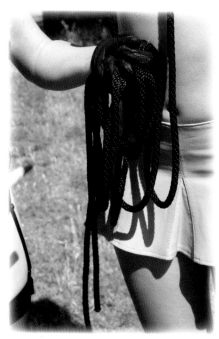

Keep ropes, lines and reins neatly folded in the hands at all times.

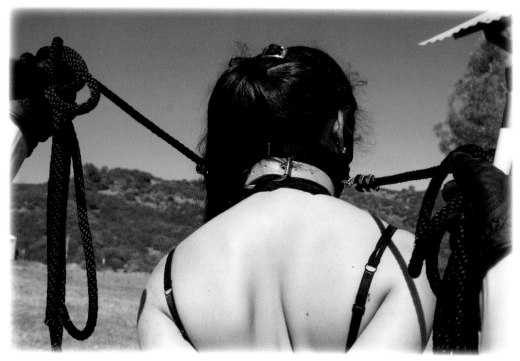

Here, the pressure is primarily on the right rein, with a 22-degree window open from 90 degrees to 112 degrees – approximately an eighth of a turn to the right.

My name is Ronin, and I love being a pony. I play as a role-play, cart, show, fetish, BDSM, and sex pony, and each aspect of pony play holds a joy for me that is different from the others.

Role-play pony headspace is different from other types of BDSM headspace. As a pony, my desires are simple: food, water, comfort and company. As a pony, I do not speak English, nor am I so good at understanding it. Yet I am confident in what I am, self-aware without being self-conscious.

When I am a cart pony, I am a beast of burden. I am useful and indispensable, for who would pull the cart but a pony?

As a show pony, I get to show off and strut my stuff. That's a lot of fun, of course – but I also get to help the human on the other end of the reins. I don't know why they want me to do what it is that they want me to do, but I do know that they want me to do it. I want to help, so I will do what they ask. To be a pony is to be the ultimate helper.

I am also a fetish pony. I love to dress up and look the part. Since I have an affinity for latex, I like to put on either a rubber catsuit or latex shorts. I also love wearing masks, and have a very nice horse head mask made of leather. And of course I love having a tail. When I wear the costume, especially the mask, it is easier for me to switch into the Ronin-the-pony persona. Also, when I wear the costume and look the part, I get a lot of positive attention at parties and gatherings. That positive attention is very nice.

As a BDSM pony, I love to have my hands bound or in hooves, my arms chained together behind my back and the bit in my mouth. I need assistance to put on my hooves,

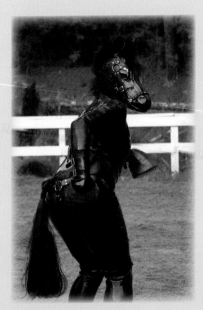

chain my arms together, and finally to put the bit in my mouth. This ritual helps to create a connection between me and my trainer/handler. Once that bit is placed in my mouth, the switch to pony space becomes almost automatic.

I am also a sex pony. I'm grinning as I type this.

I love being each type of pony, but I love being a role-play pony best. I love to act, and so I derive the joy of performance from pony play. There is more to it than that, however, as I also love to immerse myself in the role. This means that I can sometimes forget my worries in the "real world" and simply be, as a horse. This is my ultimate goal, and all else is secondary. My primary goal and reward for pony play is the reduction of the world – from bills, worries, fears, and doubts to walk, trot, left, right, stop, and carrot (yum!).

– Ronin

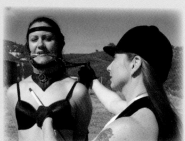

Training Tip

The natural progression of cues until the desired behavior presents:

Ask for it. Ask for it again.

Ask for it and reinforce it with an additional cue (audio, visual, physical).

Ask again, perhaps more clearly.

Clarify communication, get the pony's attention and ask again. If the pony is not doing as you ask, be sure to take into consideration the possibility of a safety issue or unaddressed need.

Increase the assertiveness of the cue by adding a training aid, such as tapping the whip on the body part of the pony that most makes sense. The pony should move away from the pressure of the cue.

The assertiveness and training aid application increase in severity. However, it may be more productive and less frustrating to the pony to try another tactic if the chosen methods don't produce results.

setting. Does it run off at the first opportunity? Does it nuzzle other ponies or stand off by itself? Is the pony polite with others? Does it get into trouble? Does it get in the way? What does the pony do when alone? Does it get into the trash, smell objects or otherwise explore its surroundings? These character and personality traits influence how the pony behaves in the community as well as in other situations. Its natural way of being with others when not under specific guidance gives the trainer an idea about how to interact with and handle the pony for training.

Deciphering character behaviors becomes easier with practice, and facilitates deeper understanding of the pony. Good understanding leads to a closer relationship with clear communication. Both increase the fun and success of a play session. The interaction unfolds naturally as the pony responds to others, both in a basic communication system and then later within the training situation.

In the biological equine world they talk about "ground manners." This term refers to how the horse behaves while the handler or trainer is "on the ground," next to the trainer, as opposed to being ridden. Trainers and handlers desire a "good," polite pony with manners, one that respects people. The "naughty" pony exhibits behavior such as kicking, biting or other forms of aggression or resistance. Effective training increases the desired behaviors and decreases the undesired behaviors through management of the pony's environment.

In-Hand Behavior. In-hand behavior implies direct contact, with the lead line, reins, and possibly other forms of bondage tethering the pony to the handler or trainer. This activity prevails in the human pony play world for practical reasons.

As the "head pony," or dominant equine, in the pony's perspective, the trainer establishes his or her personal space. This begins to define the pony's use of space. Each person who works with the pony must execute consistent handling, or bad habits will develop. A training aid such as a whip or coiled rope aids in maintaining spatial awareness. The training aid keeps the pony's attention. It is not used for impact or pain. The trainer merely taps the pony with the training aid if it gets too close. This helps teach the pony boundaries. The pony responds to commands while being guided by hand through the use of tack or training aids. Whether in the community or in hand, the pony must respect personal space; otherwise, it may overrun and possibly injure those around it.

Considering these issues ahead of time keeps the pony from learning bad habits. The human-pony community takes care of its own when it comes to expected behaviors during events and

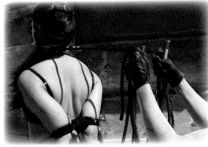
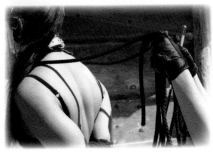

More or less tension in the reins conveys very different messages to the alert pony.

group activities. The rules of polite company apply. Desired pony behaviors include respecting unknown beings, particularly humans; friendly interactions with other ponies and animals; lack of fear; and generally a relaxed, confident manner. Training, experience and trust in the trainer develop this relaxed confidence. Poor manners include letting the pony bite others, or otherwise harm or interfere with other players. A naughty pony may need a lot of guidance. Overall consideration of the environment fine-tunes the play.

Effective in-hand training comes from clear intent. As the largest area of training for human ponies, solid in-hand work will lay the foundation for good habits when the training becomes more complex.

The pony pays attention if the trainer focuses on the pony and presents an energetic posture. The pony responds to posture and attention, learning cues by association. The trainer's signals designating relaxed mode, training mode or performance mode can be very useful in comforting the eager-to-please pony. Shortening the line between the hand and bit in order to get a slight amount of tension or connection between the hand and bit communicates the trainer's readiness to work. A whip at the ready supports the cue as a secondary cue, or training aid.

Basic common sense works for most training situations when broken down into simple elements. The rich tradition of handling biological equines also offers a wealth of information. According to tradition, the handler walks with the pony on the right (horses generally train on the right and dogs on the left). Be sure that any reins or lines are folded neatly in the hands at all times so they do not become tangled, obstructive to the training or dangerous. Keep harnesses, tack and various restraints well maintained, safe and mindful of the present effect on the pony. Be aware of the mindset, safety and general needs of the pony at all times. Good handlers or trainers only use training aids that they understand and use proficiently. Awareness of the environment, including but not limited to weather, hazards, people, animals, and obstacles, keeps everyone safer. Most importantly, a good handler or trainer projects a confident pisture, letting the pony know that the handler or trainer is in control. The trainer communicates confidence when talking to the pony calmly and directly and by only making movements with concise meaning, even when not feeling confident. Random movements and half-delivered cues confuse the pony, making it difficult for the pony to pay attention. Therefore, the trainer must first train herself by paying attention and planning ahead. Most of the general behaviors develop in both the trainer and pony as the relationship develops.

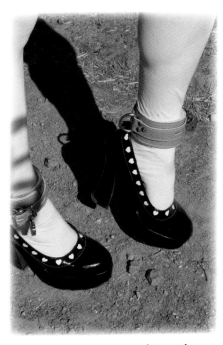

Copper paws the ground to get her trainer's attention.

Training to a Discipline. The third type of behavior deals with the pony's response to commands outside of the in-hand work. The biological equine world talks about training horses "under saddle" or "to cart" or to some other discipline, which distinguishes between the various modes of working the horse.

One way to reference the differences relates to the proximity of the work. Voice commands, direct commands, riding cues or cues from a distance all demonstrate control from a different position or distance between the handler and pony. This gets a little confusing when distinguishing between types of human pony play, due to the close proximity in general. Pony players best define the specific discipline they want to achieve for themselves.

Regardless of the activity, the training objective is to decrease the number of unwanted behaviors and increase the number of desired behaviors. The philosophies and methods of training present unlimited choices from other disciplines both inside and outside the biological equine world.

One valuable philosophy rewards the desired behaviors and controls the environment so that the only choice available elicits the desired behavior. This reward-based technique, simplifies the early days of training if used efficiently. At the more advanced stages of training, opportunities to choose the correct behavior over an incorrect choice presents the pony constructive challenges that enrich the training level. An advanced level of training has been achieved when the pony obeys the commands of the trainer regardless of personal desire. The efficient trainer learns to use the pony's motivations to meet the ends desired by the trainer; early on the pony may be motivated by treats, and later be more motivated by praise.

The trash can foraging example illustrates this concept. If the trainer wants the pony to avoid rummaging around in the trash can (yes, some human ponies rummage in the trash can) and come to her for treats, the behavior can be changed fairly easy by enclosing the pony in an area with the trash can, the trainer,and treats and/or praise. When the pony approaches the trash can the trainer uses a verbal command, body language and/or noise to mean "no." The trainer decides what word, signal, sound or combination of cues to use. Consistency makes all the difference for efficient and effective training. Usually the pony looks at the source of the "no" command in response to its foraging. The trainer grabs this opportunity to present the reward. Some trainers choose to use a treat, though verbal praise and petting work too. Most importantly, the pony builds an understanding of what the alpha pony (trainer) commands through consistent repetition.

The trainer or handler must establish herself as the dominant horse in the herd of two. Working with the idea of predator and prey as the trainer-pony relationship develops gives credibility to the play. Whether the relationship identifies as D/S based or not, the element of control by the trainer is still present. The intensity of that tone synchronizes in rhythm with the basis of the relationship. How does the trainer-as-predator gain the trust of the pony, a prey animal? Establishing trust through caring for the pony's needs works on the human level; careful attention must be paid to the needs of the pony.

If you're still confused about training language, think about opening a window. The trainer communicates a single behavior choice for the pony by constructing a closed environment with only one opening. For example, if the trainer wants the pony to turn right, the trainer makes sure the lines of the reins only allow a right turn and only to the degree desired. That means the trainer controls the reins well enough to allow only a specific range of movement. The pony doesn't have to think – she only walks through the window.

Making the right choice provides the reward in itself. Praise reinforces the right choice. Treats

---

Training Tip

To keep pony in headspace during training, disallow verbal communication except in the case of an emergency. The pony can effectively communicate a problem by simply stopping, by pawing the ground or through many non-verbal behaviors. The pony can communicate thirst by walking over to a water source and nuzzling it. Biological equines communicate their needs just fine – so can human ponies. The trainer just has to pay attention.

work well at the start of training, but ponies respond to praise just as well – if not better – within an established relationship. Later in training, the treats may distract from the attention necessary for learning or compromise the pony's health.

The trainer holds the space, both headspace and play space, for all players involved. The pony has responsibility to maintain headspace as well, but the trainer by definition leads the process. If the play space takes place in a crowded, public area, the responsibility to maintain a safe space rests even more emphatically upon the trainer.

The trainer communicates the specific needs of the pair, which may include space requirements and directives regarding touch, to the general public. That objective, clear-headed common sense, "horse sense," comes in handy during pony play. Interest and passion fuel the scene and gauge the intensity. Respect of the pony and the play itself brings integrity to the play as well as increasing safety. Keep in mind that the degree of the clarity of goals usually corresponds to the degree of success of the scene.

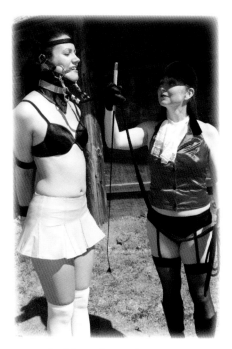

A whip at the ready acts as a secondary visual cue.

Clarity helps the pony trust the trainer within the situation as well as guiding the trainer's plan. Even if the trainer's understanding lacks clarity, the pony needs to think the trainer knows what she is doing. Clarity keeps the pony from getting confused, scared or losing respect for the trainer. Ponies need confidence and grounded energy in their trainer in order to let go of self-preservation thinking and focus on the task at hoof.

The C's of communication skills – Clear, Concrete, Consistent, Concise and Compassionate – guide the trainer in clarifying the communication in scene. When the trainer develops a plan for the session, he or she creates the road map including beginning, middle, and end/goal. The road map keeps the session on target so that the goal and the means fall into place fluidly. The better the plan the less likely the players are to get lost, the less frequently frustrations manifest, the more time for fun, and the greater the likelihood that everyone involved will enjoy themselves.

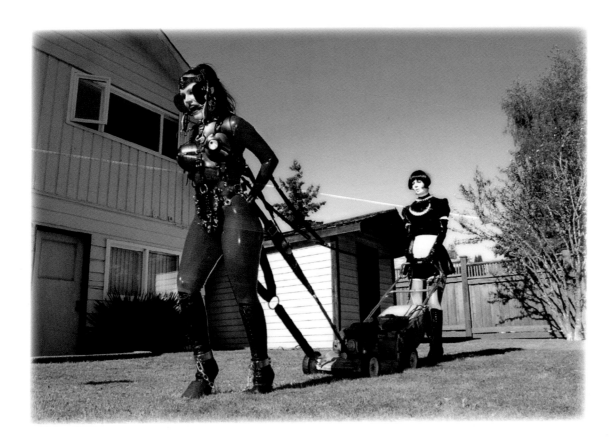

The Rodeo

So, we still hadn't figured it out. What kind of pony was my Pony? Like a good farm horse, he was helpful, useful, and strong, and he loved to take his Mistress on scenic cart rides – but I couldn't imagine him just plodding around on a field all day. And while he loved showing off new gaits and getting attention, he wasn't a fussy Arabian show pony, either. He was something more in the middle, but I wasn't sure exactly what. Then it came to me.

I had seen my first rodeo in Grass Valley, California, several years earlier. Having grown up in the East Coast, it was about as alien to me as Mars. You mean, there are real cowboys, not just the models in Marlboro ads? Yep. And they really do wear those fringed chaps, get tossed around like rag dolls by bucking broncos, and wrestle bulls to the ground. It is really quite a sight. There were even real cowgirls, leaping from one horse to another, doing handstands on the horse's backs, hanging from only one stirrup, and doing other crazy stunts. I decided that my Pony had to see this, so I took him to the Rodeo. It was kind of a surprise. This one was indoors, and there were no hand-standing cowgirls, but plenty of talented cowboys, horses, livestock and even sheepdogs. The show was incredible, especially the bronc riding, both saddle and bareback. Some of the horses just sprang straight up into the air, like they had rocket-boosters in their forelocks. Did you know they get points for how well they buck?

This rodeo also had quarter horses, a breed I thought might be a match for my Pony due to their calm temperament and helpful nature. I wasn't sure yet if it they were special enough, but the show soon changed my mind. First, we watched as two of them corralled a powerful bull calf into a pen, predicting its every move, despite the fact that it was charging in erratic zigzags all around the ring. Then, in a more formal equestrian performance, we saw their incredible agility as they trotted in impossibly tight circles and then walked effortlessly backwards. But the most dramatic move of all was this: barreling down the center of the ring at full speed, a horse went straight for us, dust flying, nostrils flared, seemingly about to run smack into the ring wall or, more likely, catapult right beyond it into our laps. And then he stopped on a dime. His entire rump came down, putting on the brakes in a cloud of dust. But the feat didn't end there. He leaped back up, spun around and rocketed to the other side of the ring, only to perform the same miraculous stop, and somehow with grace. Wow. That did it. We knew what my Pony was. (Not long after that, I taught the Pony to do all of these things, ground driving. True to his breed, he was a fast learner, and picked them up in no time.)

As soon as we got home from the Rodeo, we wanted to try everything. Especially the bucking, but since it seemed to have a pretty high potential for injury, we decided to start slow, and on something soft. I mounted bareback and without reins, but even when he bucked lightly, I would start to fall. I needed something to hold onto. Even the

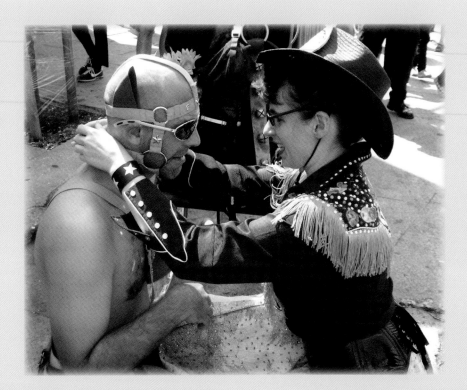

bareback riders had a nice sturdy handle to grip. So we tried strapping a strong leather belt around him and buckling it tightly at his chest, so it wouldn't move. I held on to it with one hand and raised my other arm high in the air, just like the cowboys. This time he had to work much harder to throw me. I got a good long ride before I fell off again, flopping to the side. The Pony was a good bucker, raising up and bearing down, and it was really fun.

We had our first opportunity to show off our new tricks when we were invited to perform at the annual Dog and Pony Show. The workshop presenter acted as buzzer and announcer, calling out the seconds just how they did at the Rodeo. "And they're out of the chute!! One! Two! Three! Four! Five... Bahhhhhhhhhh!" The Pony went all out, popping up like a cork, throwing out his front and hind legs, jerking his hindquarters and tossing his head. What a show-stopper! Still I held on (with only one hand, of course). We did three rounds and I managed to stay the full time for two of them, but for one he managed to throw me off, hard, and I went flying right over his head! I spun and landed completely sprawled out on the ground, breathless and laughing.* People were amused, amazed and a little bit terrified... just like the Rodeo. It was great.

Yep. My Pony was a quarter horse, and a rodeo horse to boot. He'd done me proud.

– Juliana Switch

Don't try this at home, boys and girls. And if you do anyway, don't go pointing your sprained wrists at me afterwards.

Chapter Five
Scene Development

First decide on the long term and short term goals for this particular pony, then plan the individual steps to those goals, including what commands, or cues, to use to ask for the desired behaviors. When it comes time to train the pony, the pony needs to know the language. In order to accomplish complex behaviors like driving, reining or dressage, the pony must know the commands and the steps that lead up to each of the desired behaviors – beginning from the simple and building up to the more complex. Therefore, it makes sense to teach the commands first as the training unfolds.

Common cues:
- Whistling – calling pony
- Patting – letting pony know you are there and everything is okay
- Scratching – affection
- Pushing – move over
- Clicking tongue – move out (at walk)

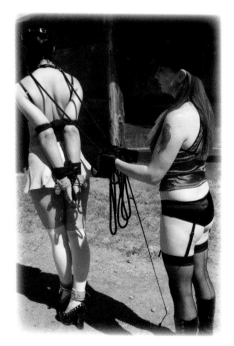

In England the ponies cross their legs when they have to go to the bathroom. Establish a cue regarding facility use ahead of time.

- Clucking/Kissing – move out with more energy
- "Ho" or "Halt"– stop
- "Walk" or "Walk on" – amble, walk out
- "Trot/Jog" – jogging pace
- "Canter/Lope" or "Hup" – gentle run with one leg leading: right or left "lead." (It's the gait children use to run like a horse. The lead is the leg in front.)
- "Run/Gallop" – full out speed
- "Step Up" – pick foot up over obstacles
- "Easy" – slow down or settle down
- "Out" – move farther away from trainer
- "High Step" – parade or pony step (Choose one variation and stick with it.)
- "Hoof" – pick up hoof to be inspected
- "Extend" – make the gait bigger, longer
- "Slow" – slow down, make the gait smaller

Each cue to behavior association must be taught. Just stay with the same cues for each pony. Ask experienced ponies for their cue preference.

Start out small and develop the play in alignment with each player's level of confidence and experience. The play expands accordingly. Effective communication makes the training process easier, which takes time and dedication to build thorough understanding. The trainer usually appreciates not having to be a mind reader and not having to guess so much, and the pony tries harder for the trainer as well. This willingness reflects the desire to please that many ponies possess. There seems to be more success in the play when the pony and trainer take the time to know each other both as players and as people in order to determine the play parameters.

Bridling, leading and establishing verbal cues with the pony make for a good start to training. Make sure to solve any tack problems ahead of training time by trying the gear on the pony before play. Biological equine trainers do this, or use specifically designed training gear for unbroken horses. Comfortable tack helps ensure that play can continue as long as desired. Keeping play simple and pleasant during training helps to maintain positive associations for both players.

Some conventions simply exhibit tradition and add credibility to the play, such as teaching the pony to walk on the right side of the trainer; other behaviors are essential for advancing the play. When executing a simple walk, if the pony gets ahead of the trainer, the trainer merely has to change directions so that the pony has to follow. Using an incentive to encourage the pony to go forward assists in urging the reluctant pony forward. Role-playing ponies often appreciate treats such as carrots, sugar cubes, candied nuts or chocolate cake for reward or motivation. An SM pony might respond better to a whip. Never confuse the two. The play might just end forever. Research the traditions of specific disciplines to expand the play over time. "Boarding," for example, cues the pony to prepare for the cart to be loaded.

Pony play scene development follows the same protocol as regular BDSM scene development. It follows a logical pattern: negotiate, establish headspace, warm up, training session

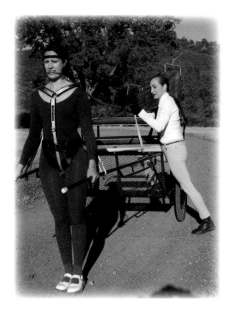

"Boarding" is the command that cues the pony to prepare for the cart to be loaded.

"We're going to a special event today," says Madam. It must be special because she has on a new tailored outfit that is very shiny. The sun reflects off it. I am so honored to pull her in the small riding cart. I am beaming. I am a lucky pony. Madam is smiling ear to ear. I can tell she is very pleased with her outfit; it was made for our event today.

I do not have to wear a modesty covering today. It will be permissible to wear my bridle and harness in my own skin in public. My hair is braided neatly and the end of my braid hangs on my back. We will use the small metal bit, a snaffle bit, in my bridle with the pretty rhinestone studded reins. I like the slender metal bit much more than the thick rubber bit piece in my mouth. It is a very sunny morning, so my eyes are protected with shades. My tail is brushed and sways over my hindquarters. Madam inspects me to make sure everything is to her liking before we enter the fair. We are stopped just outside of the side street entry gate.

I raise my leg high and stamp it down to show my excitement. "My Beauty wants to run," Madam Wilcox laughs. I must be patient. Madam has another pet, a dog, with us today. He is a handsome creature. Madam says he will be our guide dog today. The dog's name is Spike. Madam Wilcox introduces us. He is friendly and a very handsome dog. I like his head and paws very much. They are black leather. Spike is a very good and useful pet. I am glad he is here.

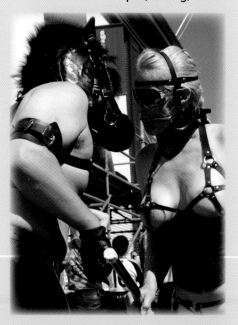

"Boarding." That is the signal for me to know that she is boarding the cart. I stand very still, holding the cart level for her. On the wide open street I am given free rein to gallop. It is all so thrilling. This is very different from our rides in the park. There are new sounds, and there is much activity on the cross street in front of us. I feel the gentle pulling back on the rein with the command to slow and I obey. Spike comes in front of me and walks about six feet in front of me. I am turned right onto the busy street.

I have never seen such things. My eyes go wide taking it all in. There is music all around. There is the sound of people talking, lots of talking so that you can't hear the words exactly. Many people are dressed in leather and they line the streets. I like the smell of leather. People are naked.

I walk, lifting my legs very high, and look ahead of me. I sense many people stopping, turning, and looking at us. I want to keep the cart level for Madam Wilcox. I am directed behind the dog. There is a commotion around me. Many people are shouting at Madam. She signals me to stop. Clicking sounds go off all around me as people form a semi-circle in front of me, and they are looking at us. The clicks are people taking pictures on their cameras. I wait patiently.

The reins jump lightly on my back and I am commanded to move. There is lots of activity around me. There are people milling about, people following us, people clicking cameras at us. Someone calls out. I smell food. The dog is waving his paws and directing people apart and we are slowly going forward. There is a crowd of people at a stand and we move slowly around them. Then I hear my driver, "Whoa." And my reins are pulled back. I stand at attention. There is a flurry of activity around us. People are talking to Madam Wilcox. I gaze out around me, taking in the attention.

Madam Wilcox is there beside me. She is smiling. She asks how I am, pats me, straightens my shades and offers me water to drink. I am a much loved pony. I get all the water I want. We are there quite a bit. I shake my head, stamp my foot, I want to pull the cart with my driver. I hear her laugh. "Are you getting impatient, Beauty?" I neigh at her: "Yes, yes, let us be off, please."

The Folsom Street Fair is very big. To my surprise there is another pony. A pretty black pony with a plume in her headdress is coming closer to us. She wears a beautiful leather harness. As her trainer brings her forward I can see and smell her better. I know her. I rub my head against her shoulder and head. I'm very happy to see her. She is very proud to be out and about with her trainer. She isn't pulling a cart, for she is dressed in fine plumage and harness, she is a show pony. There is more clicking all around us as people take pictures of the show pony and me. Everyone has big smiles.

As we continue down the street, we stop often to have a picture taken with some nice person who asks Madam. I concentrate on being mindful of the cart, be pleasant, quiet, turn as my driver wants me to, doing anything my driver wishes, focusing on where I am being directed by my reins, stepping high and properly for my driver. The street is becoming more and more full of life.

Suddenly from the sidewalk a Stud Pony prances up. He is very handsome, and shows himself off to me. I neigh back at him as Madam signals to stop. People gather around us to take more pictures. The handsome Stud Pony and I flirt with one another.

"Okay, Beauty, we must be going on, it is time for us to be finishing. The street is becoming much too busy and crowded for us." We are off again. I am allowed to gallop, pulling the cart and Madam the length of the side street. I am spent in the hot sun.

Madam dismounts the cart. She brings me water and pats me. She gives me lots of affection and tells me what a well-mannered, non-fretful and joyful pony I am. I smile as she praises the guide dog. I thank him also. I would never have been able to work my way through the crowds of people on the busy street without him.

Such a wonderful excursion we had at the Folsom Street Fair 2007. I am a very lucky pony.

– Beauty, www.submissann.com

and cool-down or aftercare. The scenarios change but the pattern remains the same.

Negotiations for a one-time shot at a hot scene must address in detail the capabilities and expectations of each player before entering head space. Remember that after entering headspace, the ability to make appropriate decisions decreases. Luckily for new trainers, human ponies have human brains under their pony brains that they can use for communication when necessary.

Within the parameters of a long-term relationship, time allows development of a long term training plan for "breaking in" the pony and training it step by step to do complex behaviors.

Suggested hierarchy of training lessons:

- Develop partnership/relationship
- Develop trust and bonding
- Teach pony to accept gear willingly
- Groom pony
- Teach pony to lead

Training Tip

Handlers and trainers must keep in mind that the pony might not be able to make good decisions for himself when in pony headspace. One pony told a story of how she went into sugar overload and later crashed because she was fed too many sugar cubes. The handler, who knew about the pony's sugar sensitivity, gave permission for a bystander to offer a sugar cube in a public situation. For this pony, one cube would have been fine. However, the bystander fed the pony a second sugar cube without the handler's knowledge. The pony normally adhered to her dietary requirements when using her human brain to say "no." However, while under the influence of pony headspace, she ate the sugar cube because it tasted good. The depth of the headspace amazed the pony in retrospect: she normally makes safe and healthy choices. Trainers and handlers are advised to know each pony's specifics and health requirements and to be aware that bystanders can profoundly affect the well-being of the pony, however unintentionally.

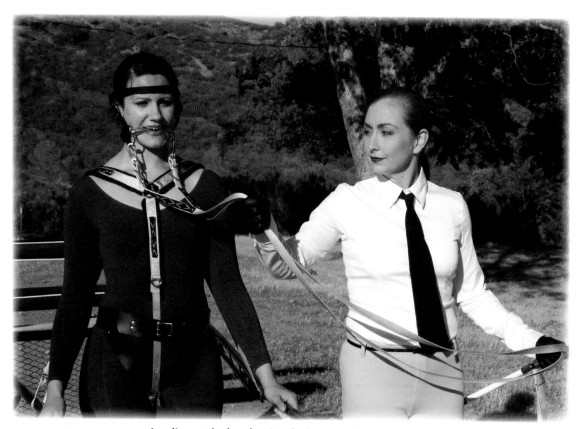

Leading at the head trains the intermediate pony to cart.

- Teach pony basic in-hand cues – no, stand, forward, back, over, respect your space, etc.– as well as general manners
- Gaits
- Lunging
- Ground driving
- Specific discipline according to type of play

Here is an example of a training hierarchy using cart play as the discipline. Other discipline options might include jumping, obstacles, reining, pulling work loads, events, show and so on.

- Harnessing up to the cart
- Lead at head with cart
- Ground drive with cart
- Drive from cart

Training Tip

Ponies go where their heads are turned and to the degree they are turned. A soft turn to the right requires a soft pull on the right rein (or pull softly on the lead rope to the right). The strength, speed, and intensity of the pull determines the degree and speed of the turn. Most human ponies require light tension on the rein. In fact human necks, particularly those with past injuries, necessitate great care. Pull gently until the pony's head points in the direction requested of the pony, and then just keep the reins solidly in place. Sometimes the pony tries too hard and turns back and forth. Keeping the reins gently taut and in place opens the window by allowing only the right choice. Sometimes the pony needs to be encouraged to move forward through the open window by the trainer giving a cue to do so, such as a verbal "walk-on" or tap on the rump with a whip. For ponies who think too much about other things while playing, a simple directive (offered to the human in advance of the play) to "go where your head is pointed" helps. If the pony anticipates the cue and turns too far, the trainer needs to change the activity in order to get the pony's attention, either by changing the pace or altering the pattern. Making decisions regarding training techniques becomes easier with experience.

Supplemental Training Lessons:

- Coordination
- Obedience
- Conditioning
- Agility, fluidity
- Obstacles
- Socialization

The owner, trainer, or handler takes responsibility for the care and edification of the pony. Regardless of the relationship, whoever handles the pony has a responsibility to create a safe physical, mental and emotional environment. Headspace merely covers one aspect to the reason of this responsibility. It also includes the implied and actual control of the handler over the pony, particularly in regard to the bondage aspects of the play. The handler takes on the real and implied caregiver role. Within the context of play, the trainer must think for the pony, even if the pony is very smart, as well as keeping an eye on the pony's bondage and environment. Not only does the trainer need to monitor all aspects of the play, but he also needs to think three steps ahead in the scene in order to progress with the training sequence.

That seems like mental juggling in the beginning. In order to accomplish it, the trainer must first know himself and the pony. Secondly, the trainer must know the plan for the training session; having even a general goal assists in sustaining a proper training session. Thirdly, the trainer must consider the environment, including any change in the pony's headspace or well-being, and change the training plan as needed to adapt to the situation.

If the pony shows undue or unplanned distress during the training session, stop the activity immediately and go back a step or two in the training sequence. A familiar situation reassures the pony, enabling the play to continue without a negative experience. From that point, the trainer evaluates how to proceed, perhaps by trying again, changing the cues, or ending on a good note. First, assume the pony wants to obey, even if it's a "naughty" pony (exceptions might include negotiated resistance and/or cathartic play), and thus err on the side of caution. Ponies generally strive to please their trainers and respond sensibly. Acting up, or refusing a cue, frequently derives from a very good reason. A leg caught in the lunge line or an ill-fitting piece of equipment might cause the resistant behavior. Hunger, thirst or other needs cause distraction. If the pony is disobedient, use reasoning skills to discover the cause

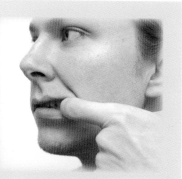

Try It

Put your finger in the corner of your mouth and gently pull back. Notice how little pressure it takes to affect your head. Players commonly use too much pressure in the beginning. Less is more. When in doubt, back off. The positive association supersedes the possibility of going too far.

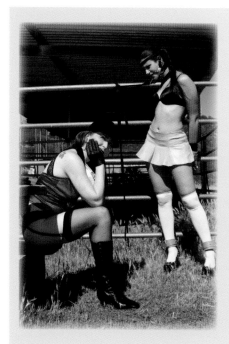

Training Tip

If you begin to lose control, stop. The pony's safety is at risk. Tie the pony up, turn it loose for a bit, give it to someone else for a minute, or choose something more appropriate to the play scenario. Providing a time-out gives the pony time to relax and protects the pony from confusion caused by the erratic behavior of the trainer. The trainer can then decide how best to continue after some time to calm down and reflect. Continuing play allows for a positive association to continue. If the play stops altogether on a negative note, a negative association may be built between the pony and the training sessions or trainer. Always find a way to end on a good note.

An Example of an Intermediate Scene

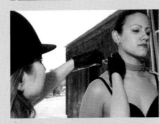

.... Capture the pony

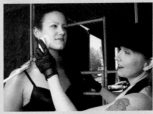

.... Tie the pony in cross ties

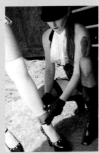

.... Groom the pony

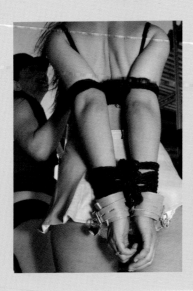

.... Tack

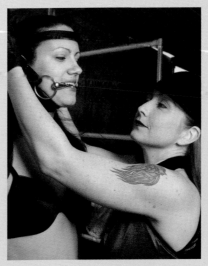

Tacked up and
ready to go!

Warm up with lunging or ground driving ....

Left turn while driving on long lines ....

Hitch up to a cart...

Drive..

Unhitch...

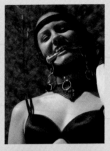

.... Reward and thank pony

Walk out pony by hand for cool down

Groom/check pony

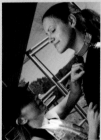

.... Blanket pony to keep muscles from cooling off too fast

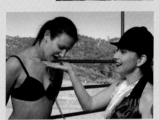

.... Light water and snacks

of the distress. The handler entertains several possibilities for the cause of poor behavior at the same time, all the while maintaining clear communication with the pony. Multi-tasking becomes a way of being for the trainer.

Confidence comes in handy too. If the trainer communicates ambiguous cues during the exploration of the situation, confusion generally ensues. If the pony performs a behavior other than what the trainer asked for, the trainer will do well to assume that the communication failed somehow, rather than jump to the conclusion that the pony misbehaved on purpose. When in doubt, stop and regroup. The motivations for the seemingly random

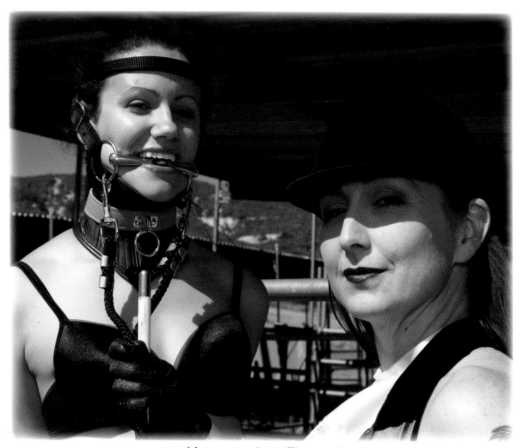

A happy pony is a willing pony!

behavior of the pony will be more clear to the trainer as pony and trainer continue to play.

Lunging presents a fun opportunity for training, conditioning and play. To teach the pony to lunge, first review the voice commands for walk, trot, canter, high step, extend, slow, ho, back, stand and out, or other specific commands necessary. The trainer begins by planting a heel at the center of the circle and then asks the pony to "walk-on." Little by little the rein or rope releases while the trainer taps the pony, nudging the pony toward the outer edge of the circle, while saying "out." The whip helps to cue the pony to move out on the circle. The trainer remains on the inside of the circle in one place as the pony moves out on the edge

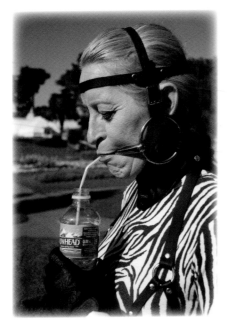

**Remember to offer snacks
and water frequently.**

of the circle. The length of the rein determines the radius. A long whip of some kind cues the pony from a distance when necessary. A slight tap with the whip reinforces "out" or "ho" when held out in front of the pony. Practice "ho" and "walk" until both pony and trainer feel comfortable and sure of the footing. The pony requires work in both directions in order to remain balanced. Human ponies ordinarily find the second side easier. Practice all the gaits and commands in both directions, keeping it easy and simple by adding just one new thing at a time. Lunging develops endurance and practice for the pony without tiring the trainer.

General Cautions...

- Be mindful of the pony's headspace.

- Actively look for hazards.

- If you take your pony in public be sure you pre-negotiate approval for petting, pictures, etc.

- Think about the pony's physical needs: keep the pony hydrated and blood sugar up. Offer snacks every two to four hours and water at regular intervals, probably every thirty to sixty minutes.

- Consider the pony's emotional needs. Be respectful of your negotiated relationship with the pony and the inherent trust placed in your hands.

- Know your pony's condition level: cardio-vascular, weight training abilities, dexterity, flexibility, balance and so forth.

Pony gear is bondage:

- Bit gag – check ability to breathe and swallow.

- Arm binding – pony can't catch himself.

- Most people can't open the jaw as widely as most commercially purchased pony bits require.

- Keep in mind that increased saliva on the lips increases the dryness and cracking of the lips. Have lip balm available.

Any restraining gear – consider the effects of the following:

- Restricted mobility.

- Strain on joints.

- Decreased circulation.

Conditioning:

- Ponies may have to work up to longer and longer times of conditioning to be in the gear. Avoid muscle strain and increased tension by taking frequent breaks.

- Ponies may have to build physical endurance to perform tasks, especially for prolonged work.

- Massage helps the pony recover faster and keeps the pony happy and willing.

Head restraint:

- No jerking or sudden movements – avoid neck injury.

- If there is past history of neck problems, use voice commands only or other types of harnessing.

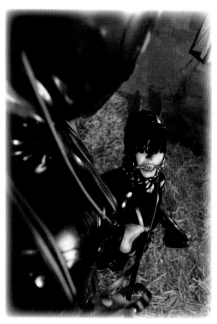

Be respectful of the inherent trust your pony places in your hands.

Even when I'm just trotting around my own bedroom, reveling in the ring of steel horseshoes against wooden floorboards, pony play seems to bring with it the smell of grass, a sense of green and the vast outdoors. Every color is brightened, every scent intensified, and conscious thought gives way to physical instinct. It's so wholesome I can't think of it as kinky, although the steel-hoofed boots I wear came from a rubberwear shop and my tail swishes from the back of a modified strap-on harness. When my trainer ties me up I'm not being put into sexual bondage (although the knots are all the same)- she's just giving me reins, correcting my posture and tucking my useless arms carefully out of the way.

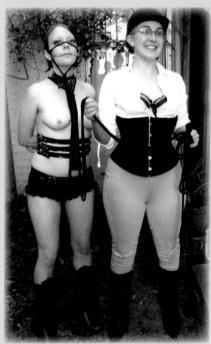

It's such a gentle transformation at her hands, from barefoot girl to head-tossing equine delight. She guides my feet into my special boots and runs her hands gently over thigh muscles that shake slightly with the strain of the exaggerated posture until every part of my body – from the balls of my feet to my shoulders – remembers that I am a pony, and adjusts. My hands disappear next, secure behind my back, and with each adjustment my sense of the world shifts markedly from words and descriptions to sound, scent and sharp color. By now I am leaning to follow her hands, letting my eyelashes flicker over her jaw and smelling the sweat behind her ears, utterly intent on her. And she is someone quite different from the good friend who comes around to play pony with me sometimes: Her smile softens, her hands become gentle, and the ringing note of pride in her voice is unmistakable. She makes me a pony and in return I make her a lady.

The final stage of the transformation is the bit slipped into my mouth – soft, bitter rubber – taking away speech and the last lingering fragment of humanity. I am forced now to communicate with my eyes and my posture, and to let my instincts guide me. We are engaged in constant conversation from here on, her with words, commands and the touch of her hands, and me with whickers, kicks and the dip of my very long eyelashes.

Preparations complete, we are able to run beautifully amok, eyes bright with the thrill of sweaty, dusty, breathless freedom. Ribbons she has braided through my tail stream and snap, bells ring, hoofs ring out a perfect rhythm. She corrects my steps and posture with sharp, clear commands, directs me with tugs of the reins, and when I get carried

"Strawberry and Miss Blonde." Photographer Joni Gear.

away and try to bolt off into the bright, distracting world, she brings me back to her with my name, called once.

When we stop for water and a brush down, the blue of her eyes and the pink of her cheeks are absolutely magical. A pony's eyes are fascinated with such details, and able to detect the slightest movement of fingers towards the pocket that holds the sugar cubes. She laughs and sighs with the liberties I take as my mouth lunges for my reward, reminds me to be gentle as I lift the sweet treat from her fingers with careful lips and crunch it down. I can smell another cube in her pocket, and try reaching my mouth out for that one too, but pushing my luck is not wise with my lady; she snaps me briskly back to attention and launches back into my training.

These hours are our time, and ours alone. For the connection to be strong and true we need this time together, for my confidence in her to be absolute and for her to know she can take the proper care of me. Because when a young lady steps out into the world with her pony on display, as my lady so loves to do, she needs to know absolutely that her pony will be a source of pride rather than worry for her. The world of people outside can be startling and stressful, full of unpredictable hazards, and a good trainer will make sure that she gives her pony the focus and grounding required to take on this unpredictable environment with calm and poise. I need not fear the world outside because I know she can take care of me in it. Her words and crop are much sharper for rough, strange hands than they ever are for me, and I know too that if I become confused she will make each bright color, unfamiliar smell, or sudden sound make sense to me.

With focus and care, our adventures outside into the world can be beautiful. I love to make her proud of me, love to hold myself tall and straight, and keep perfect time with my hooves, and I lift my chin high to show how perfectly she has groomed me for display. For the sake of her smile I am patient with every set of excitable hands that wants to pat the pony, and I am always happy to take carrot sticks and sugar cubes from unfamiliar outstretched palms as long as she's there to guide them.

It is always a relief, though, to retreat back into our close, special space, to feel her eyes on me alone and to know that nothing distracts me from her. With her hands on me, gentle and calming, we begin our slow ritual of transformation in reverse. She brushes me down, first with a spiky brush that makes my limbs burn, and then a soft glove for soothing strokes. Then she unbuckles the bit, with another carrot stick for a job well done. I can feel the world of words and human understanding start to trickle back now, as she taps my calf so I'll know to lift my hoof, which becomes a boot that she unbuckles and slips off. Standing flat my body changes, my centre of gravity lowers, and when she unties the ropes holding my hands back I am once more fully human. We stand face to face for long moments as I take in the world with human eyes, then reach with human hands to hug her to me and say "thank you" with human words.

– Ali Haberfield

- Develop a light hand using gentle cues. Think pressure, not pulling. It should only take a bending of the finger (even with a 1200-pound biological horse). The arm doesn't move.

- Sometimes ponies need their heads free from tension on the lead line or reins for safety reasons such as to negotiate stairs, check footing, relax neck muscles, etc.

- Keep reins, lead rope and lunge lines in an orderly fashion, keeping them separated, not wrapped around hands or arms, and out of the way of the pony.

- Don't secure the pony to any large object without being sure of its stability or pony's ability. For example, don't secure the pony to a cart if the pony might get too tired to hold it up and keep balance. Otherwise you might have an emergency room visit to keep you entertained instead of playing.

Consider both short-term and long- term training objectives. A written hierarchy of training lessons maintains congruence and consistency. Think through the steps necessary to achieve the final goal and what behaviors will be major performance landmarks. Each landmark breaks down into smaller pieces until the divisions create easily achievable sections for adaptation into scenes. The long term goal of training a pony to cart, for example, easily divides into multiple training scenes as the pony achieves each training landmark.

Each trainer possesses a training philosophy based on personal values. Understanding those values expressly determines the organizational level of the training plan. Beginning trainers may only address

Training Tip

Coach ponies ahead of time for particularly difficult cues or to address past miscommunications. For example, human ponies commonly overcompensate for head cues, especially before they learn how not to think like a human all the time. Ask the pony to go in the direction of the head turn. With the head turn of 30 degrees, make a slight adjustment in that direction. If the head turns 90 degrees, make a 90 degree turn. Communicate your intention of asking for the degree of the turn by the intensity of the pressure on the rein. Light pressure on the mouth/head cues a light or easy turn; increased pressure cues a more pronounced turn. This little communication saves a lot of frustration and time.

personality and general description regarding expectations of a successful scene. Spending the time developing the philosophy and training plan generally pays off in a fluid, efficient, enjoyable scene.

Once the trainer has the end in mind and decides how to proceed, then the actualization of the goals becomes more likely to manifest. How can objectives be reached without definition? If leading the pony around a campground in headspace defines success and headspace occurs with just a bit and a lead line, success comes easy. However, if success means a four pony synchronization drill team, the planning involves concentrated effort, perhaps even enlisting the help of a choreographer. The problem lies in trying to accomplish a goal in one scene that requires hours of preparation and practice. Instead, visualize the goal first, break it down and then execute the plan.

In the end, fun and personal enrichment motivate the play. The pieces come together with clear communication and planning. Even though the trainer designs the training session, planning with the pony increases the potential of matched expectations and successful interactions. Deciding on the personal application of training aids, rewards and cues that elicit the desired behaviors becomes a key element in developing the training plan.

Try-It

Practice Zen meditation to develop an open mind that allows suspension of time and desire. Learning to open the hand of thought helps both the pony and handler to be present to the play.

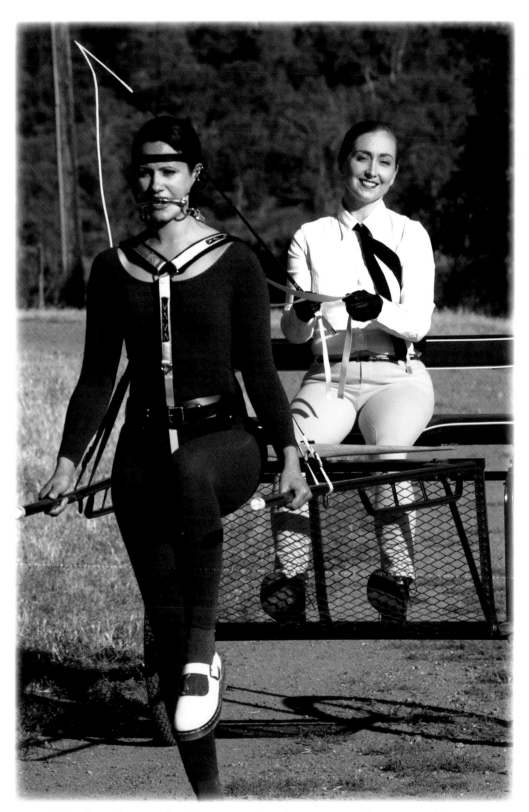

When fun and personal enrichment combine, the outcome is a happy, graceful scene.

Chapter Six
Handling and Grooming

Sometimes someone who is not a pony's trainer nonetheless handles or grooms it. Perhaps the trainer has delegated these responsibilities to another person, or perhaps he simply identifies with the role of handler or groomer. Each couple will define the boundaries between these terms differently, but in this chapter I distinguish them from one another for the sake of clarity.

Trainers allow others to handle a pony in order to give it exercise, to increase the breadth of play between the handler and pony, or to allow the trainer time to play with other ponies. When a trainer hands the pony to a handler or groom, she communicates the pony's personality, individual needs, training level, and known cues to the new caretaker. A walk-through of the commands while the trainer is still present ensures a better understanding by the handler. Of course, the trainer should know the ability of the handler and not

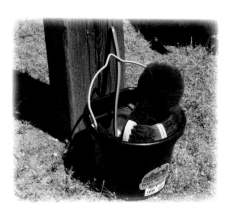

Grooming is made easy and pleasant by having all your gear ready in one place.

ask too much of her. Each player defines her role according to her individual interests and comfort.

Handling primarily refers to in-hand work, but may include putting a pony "through its paces." Putting a biological equine through its paces means going over each of the known training behaviors of the animal for evaluation, reinforcement of training or exercise. A well-trained handler repeats training lessons to further the value of the pony by increasing its ability and training level.

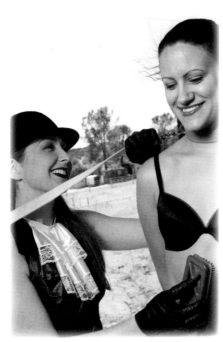

Grooming a pony refers to bathing, brushing, massaging, and generally caring for the pony's physical well-being.

Grooming a pony refers to bathing, brushing, massaging and generally caring for the pony's physical well-being. In the biological equine world, grooms attend to all areas of basic horse care, including feeding, turning out to run free in an exercise pen and monitoring health on a day to day basis. In pony role-play, the term often connotes hedonic and intimate sensation play. Preparing the pony for a fetish event or nightclub outing exemplifies a play scene where grooming and light handling may be the emphasis. This activity alone satisfies partners primarily interested in fetish or show pony play.

A fully-groomed pony presented for training or show is said to be "turned out." A properly turned-out pony exhibits a show-quality appearance, with the tack presented in a clean, attractive and safe manner. The pony also exhibits a willing disposition and a relaxed state of mind.

Grooming kits can include a broad variety of tools, especially when the primary focus is on sensation play. Many grooming tools

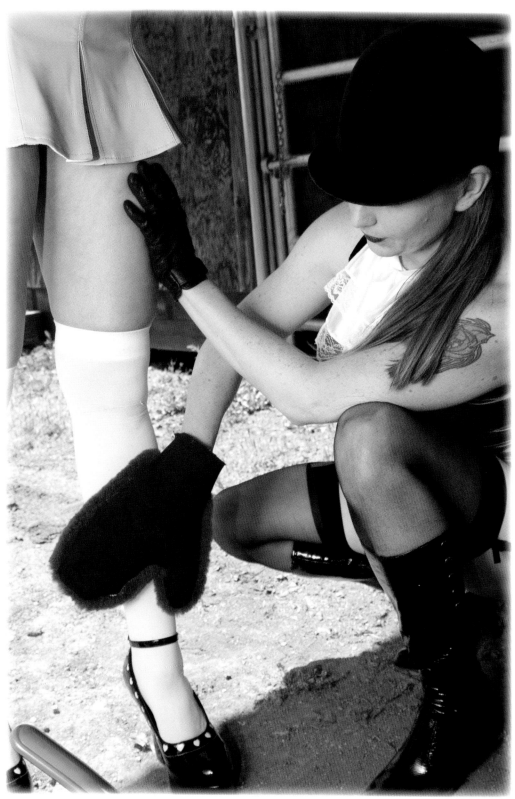

Most ponies love to be groomed.

designed for biological equines adapt well to human pony play. These can be easily acquired from on-line stores, neighborhood tack shops, and ranching stores. A good grooming kit includes a variety of sensation-delivery devices, such as a knobby "curry" tool, sometimes called a "curry comb," and a rubber bathing glove, all of which work well for human ponies. Other grooming tools include a finishing brush, a soft face brush, a comb for the mane and tail, and a hoof pick. Another option, particularly adaptable to SM play, includes a "sweat scraper."

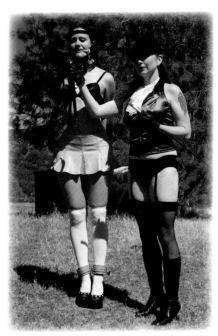

Copper turned out for show.

Even human grooming equipment translates well into a pony grooming kit. Brushes and spa products can be a decadent addition. Whatever works for the pony's pleasure and good looks is good enough. Some grooms even bathe the pony. That may translate into a anything from a sensual shower with intimate scrubbing, to a hosing off with cold water after a hard workout in the back yard.

Grooms of biological equines have no expectation of staying dry; a bathing suit at the barn works just fine. Fussy trainers frequently pawn this job off on an assistant, namely the groom.

Massage during the grooming session augments the play while communicating love for and devotion to the pony; it also generates a variety of health benefits, including but not limited to increases in circulation, relaxation, well-being, flexibility, coordination and body awareness. Ponies ordinarily love massage.

The biological equine world propagates an entertaining and wryly true inside joke: owners know they don't own the horse; on the

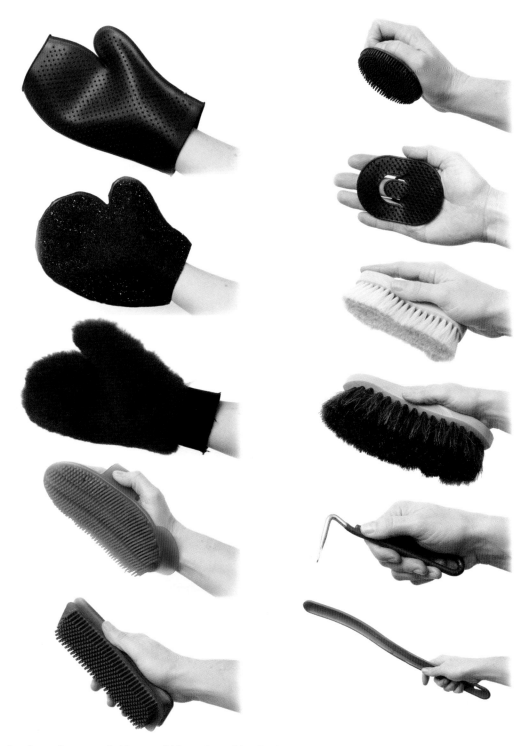

Left column from top: Rubber scrubbing mitt; rubber loofa mitt; fuzzy grooming mitt; plastic scrubbing brush, good for mane and tail too; soft rubber curry brush. Right column from top: Small curry comb; Human grooming device adaptation; small, soft facial brush – every pony's favorite; finishing brush; hoof pick for sensory/role-play; sweat scraper for wiping off water, sensory play, role play and impact play.

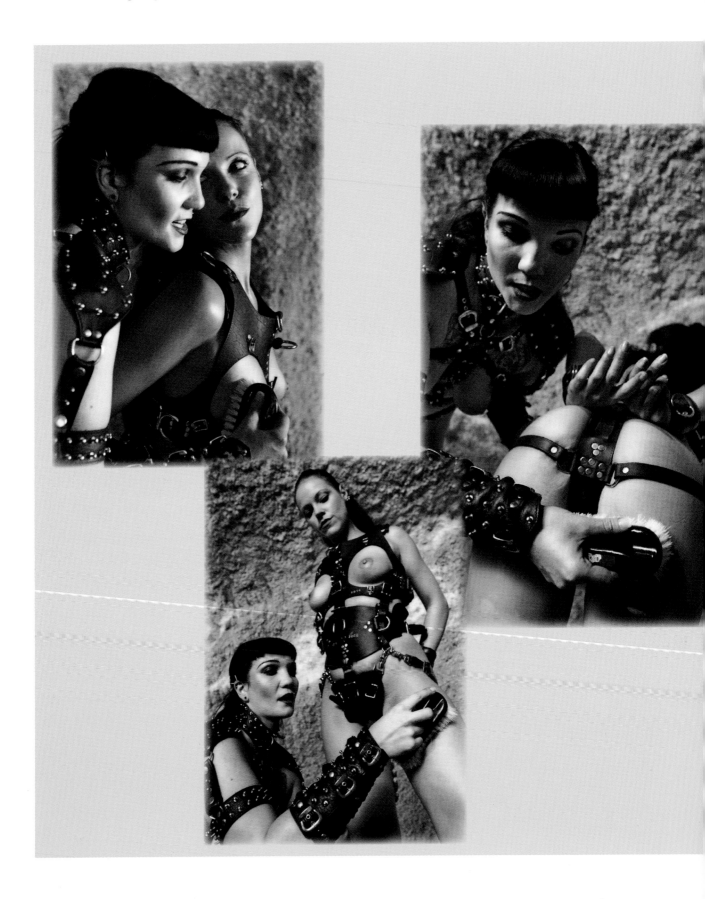

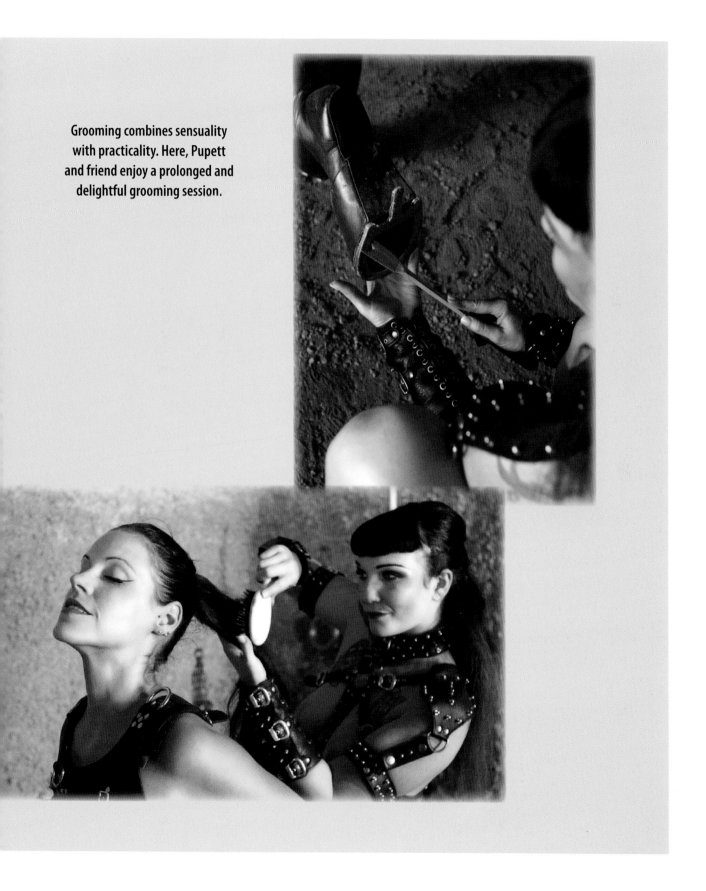

Grooming combines sensuality with practicality. Here, Pupett and friend enjoy a prolonged and delightful grooming session.

contrary, the horse actually owns them. The sentiment speaks to the time, money and love that go into caring for the equine. As with many worthwhile activities, caring for the pony requires more complexity and commitment than it seems.

If the passion to play with ponies exists, a role to play follows, even if becoming a trainer seems like too big of a task. Players have established whole training barns, from trainer to groom, with multiple ponies. Who knows? Imagination constructs the role and the possibilities therein.

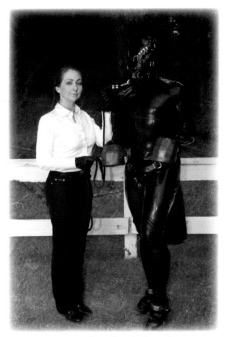

Proper in-hand or halter class technique for showing pony.

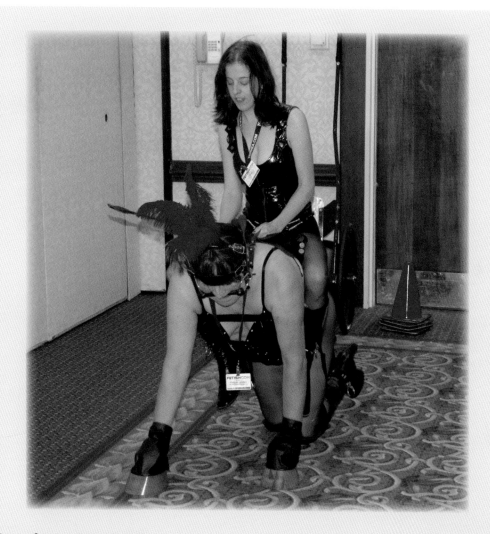

Notes from a Pony Family

Pony Lyndsey writes: As a young transsexual female, I had the joy and privilege to own my own horse. Buttercup, a beautiful white mare, was the gentlest horse I have ever known... that is, unless the person attempting to ride her was *not* me. She and I had a special attraction that I now know is probably due to the "pony" that has always been part of me.

I was quite young when I first discovered human pony play even existed. I had gotten my hands on an early BDSM publication and as I was looking through this magazine, I noticed a young lady tacked up as a pony. My initial reaction was, "Wow! You mean people do this for fun? I've got to try this someday!" After more than thirty-six years in the BDSM lifestyle, many of them as an owned/collared slave, my opportunity to "try this someday" finally came and I have not been the same woman since.

"Ponygirl Lyndsey and Hazelnut" – Photographer Keith Humphreys FSA FED

Due to circumstances that I need not expound upon here, I left my last Domme in January of 2006. After more than a year of wandering and wondering, I was sitting in the room I rented in a beautiful home on a Monday evening, alone as usual. I had recently decided that I had been keeping to myself long enough and needed to "live" again. While trying to decide what I was going to do on the weekend, I received an email from a gentleman who identified himself as Tim the Ponygroom. He mentioned that He had been reading my online profile that He had found through the membership list of one of the local munch groups that we both belong to, and had noticed that I mention pony play amongst my BDSM interests. I said that I had always been interested since I was young and had discovered human ponies. He was curious why our paths had not crossed yet and why we had not met at one of the munch events. I admitted that I had only very recently begun to pull myself out of a spell of depression.

The group was scheduled to have its monthly evening munch at a local restaurant the next Friday. Tim asked if I planned to attend. I told Him that I was on a very limited budget and did not have the funds for gasoline or to pay for my meal. Tim said, "If I can travel almost two hours to get there, you can travel for forty-five minutes to get there. You be there, and I'll see to it that you can get back home." My response: "Yes, Sir, I will be there." My life has not been the same since.

My first training session took place about two weeks after this first meeting. I was overjoyed when Ponygroom told me about halfway through the evening that there is a gentle mare inside of me. When the evening was over, we sat and talked awhile about this session and if I wanted to continue. "Oh, Sir Tim, I really do wish to learn and become the best ponygirl that I can. Please, train me, Sir. I want to be Your ponygirl full-time."

This would not be easy. At the time, we lived more than two and a half hours apart. I was unemployed, and training times had to be arranged around Tim's schedule and the ability to find places to train. As I was having no luck finding work or even getting interviews in the area where I was living, Tim suggested that I apply for jobs close to where He lived. So I did. I got an interview for every job I applied for in that area! I soon found a job in the same city, and a tiny little room only minutes from where Tim lived at the time. This room was so small Tim called it my "stall," a term that we joked about quite a bit afterwards. I was now in a position to begin Pony training, and make becoming Tim's Ponygirl a reality. We have been together now for more than six months and I have come a very long way.

I have progressed from just being a show pony to pulling our cart, and also to being ridden as a four-legged pony. As Sir tacks me up for our training session or for public showing, cart pulling, or being ridden, once my bit is in place, I am no longer Lyndsey the TS female. No longer Lyndsey the woman. I become a pony: Ponygirl lyndsey.

I respond only to the pull of the reins on the bit, or the pull on the nipple rings when they are connected to the delicate chain leads, and the short oral commands that I have been taught. To me, "pony headspace" is way different from the type of "subspace" I can and do achieve in other BDSM activities. In my subspace, I go completely out and am totally unable to respond or even safeword if needed. When in pony headspace, I am aware of the world around me, but only partially, not at all on the same level as when I am human. I do not understand English except for the verbal commands that have I been trained to respond to, nor am I totally aware of what goes on around me. I am aware if I am showing, pulling the cart, or being ridden, but time has no significance to me. I don't know how long or how many rides I may have given during that time. For instance, at a recent training session, the hosts had a dog that was quite fascinated with my ponytail and, as I have been told and seen in the pictures that were taken, loved to either follow along behind me sniffing, or, quite often, lead the way in front of me – but I don't remember this.

After a training session or a showing, I am very tired, but relaxed and thrilled that I have been a "good pony" and that I have pleased my Owner. When asked by my beloved Ponygroom if good ponies should be spanked, my response has always been, "Yes, Sir!" This sometimes leads to other BDSM activities and the opportunity to go into subspace, but that is another story.

This has been a lifelong dream of mine: to be a ponygirl. Now that I have become one of Ponygroom's ponygirls, I have joined His household stable that includes Kirby, also known as ponygirl hazelnut, who also sometimes assists in my training. The three of us are very happy to be a family and look forward to many happy, rewarding, learning, loving and blessed years together.

Hazelnut writes: I am a bondage model and a ponygirl. My groom is Tim, a.k.a Ponygroom. I had the pleasure to meet him at a play party. I witnessed him leading a volunteer around and I was curious. Afterwards, I gathered the courage to approach Tim and eagerly announced that I wanted to be a pony! He was surprised, yet pleased. He instructed me on the proper stance and gait. I pranced from one end of the house to the other with knees high and my toes pointed down. It was difficult to concentrate as I imagined how ridiculous I must appear. Gradually, however, I realized my love of being a ponygirl.

It takes ample focus for me to travel to ponyspace. One such event occurred during FetishCon 2007. I had the honor of being painted by Pashur, a body-painting artist. The body-painting process consisted of manually applying the first coat of paint and then airbrushing the second coat. Naturally, this was a tedious process, and I was uncomfortably chilled. I passed the time sporadically chatting as Ponygroom regularly checked on our progress. After I dried, I tacked up with my harness, tail, boots, headstall and bit. By that time, Ponygroom had returned; he gave me a long, light-blue shirt to cover myself in order to travel to the convention floor.

I was hustled over to a booth for a shoot. I was bound for a while as curious onlookers wandered by and eager photographers got their opportunity. This "captured pony" enjoyed the concentrated attention and the secure ropes. I struggled moderately with the bit as the drool accumulated. After a few minutes, I was released and led to another booth, where I was guided into a vertical cage. As the door closed, I was on my way into ponyspace. I recall being instructed to pose while Ponygroom explained the nature of ponies. I let myself drift away from the crowd, the noise and the motion. At one point, I was transferred to a vertical cross. After being bound there and turned horizontal, I could still hear Tim's voice, which was comforting. I am not sure when I was unbound.

I rise languidly from ponyspace as if I am underwater. I'm not burdened by petty thoughts or complicated emotions; I choose to focus instead on the movement of my body. The pressure of the bit, the tug of the reins, and Ponygroom's commands are of paramount importance. My vision narrows as I become more graceful. I have arrived at being free! Ponygroom awaits my return with patience.

I also share a stable with ponygirl lyndsey, who is an extremely hard-working pony. We frolic while we seek out tasty morsels such as bits of chocolate. As I contemplate my future training, I graciously thank Ponygroom for his love and patience.

Ponygroom writes: PonyOATS, our Florida pony play group, had been going for about a year when I found Lyndsey. For about a year I had been searching for someone who was serious about being trained. I love introducing people to the art, craft and inner life of being a pony; it's what's kept me involved in ponyplay for ten years. The demonstration sessions I had been holding, in Ocala at Sir Kane's and in south Florida at the Lifestyle Alternatives Centre of West Palm

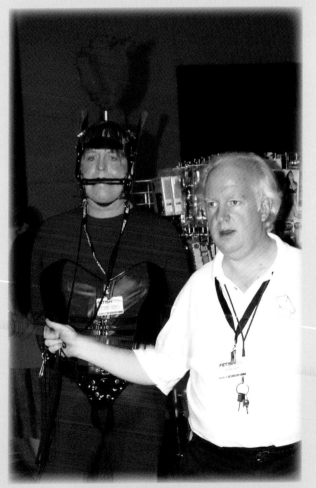

"Ponygirl Lyndsey and Ponygroom" – Photographer Keith Humphreys FSA FED

Beach, included the basic explanations followed by introducing someone to tack and training; this often resulted in a personally transformational experience for the volunteer.

I was hoping to train someone progressively. This takes commitment and a special kind of person. In Lyndsey I found such an individual.

So far, almost all of the ponies I have met who have a continuing interest in being a pony remember fondly some involvement with horses in their youth. My own time boarding a pregnant mare when I was a teenager is the wellspring of my interest.

There is something about knowing horses that inspires us. If you have never met a horse, imagine a "super pet." Brighter than dogs, often more playful than cats, horses are loyal and strong, often gentle, and sometimes wild. No two horses have the same personality. They bond to their owners. They love attention. They seek to please you; the wise human uses that instinct to train them.

I discovered in 1997 that I enjoyed relating to human horses as much as I did my pregnant mare. I saw Rogue Pony tack up at a party in Philadelphia and immediately my mind ran to how to improve her tack, and wondering if she could jump in those boots. We were already friends, but this was a different side of her I had not seen. We soon became "pony and groom," and for more than a year we went to clubs, parties and events in the mid Atlantic area. I learned a lot from her.

One of the things she taught me was that human ponies often follow patterns of behavior associated with certain breeds. For example, the stocky guy who loves to pull a cart but still stands proud in a show we think of as a Clydesdale. On the other hand, Kirby, tacked up as pony Hazelnut, is a gentle mare of no specific breed I can identify (but that may be because I don't know enough about horse breeds).

In the fall of 2006 I was at Sir Kane's place in the Ocala, Florida, area for the usual monthly PonyOATS gathering. That night, after I finished exercising pony Fayth, Kirby came up to me and said, "I want to be a pony!" This was the most direct and insistent request for training I had ever experienced! We set to work right away. Fayth's tack fit her more or less. She staggered through the basic step training as most do, but smiled all the way. Just going through the motions was getting at something in her head, something intense and personal, but I could not tell what it was right away.

Since that first experience we have had several more opportunities to train and exercise. Each time, the experience gets a little deeper for her. One of the greatest treasures of my life is the session we spent when she first experienced pony space. She had been moving stiffly, struggling to keep her balance, and obviously uncomfortable. Very suddenly she became relaxed under the reins! Her movements became fluid and graceful. I stopped her walking and went to look at her face. She had changed. I was no longer looking at Kirby: I was looking into the face of Hazelnut. We spent the next hour doing maneuvers between the traffic cones we had set up for the pony practice area, pulling the small cart and the large one, practicing the high step. She remembers very little of all that, but Hazelnut does. When we go back to training, and Hazelnut comes out to play, Hazelnut remembers her training.

Developing Hazelnut is only one of Kirby's many interests. We don't play very often, but when we do, it's a warm and wonderful experience for both of us.

In the spring of 2007, I found Lyndsey on the mailing list for the Florida Space Coast Munch. She mentioned "pony play" as an interest on her Yahoo profile. After a few online chats and emails, we talked on the phone, and then agreed to meet at the next FSC monthly munch.

A very excited and warm Lyndsey sat across from me at our table at that munch. I showed her Issue 20 of *Equus Eroticus*, the one with Fayth on the cover. I had the tack from that cover shot with me in a bag under the table. This was her first time actually touching tack; her eyes were wide with anticipation. I learned of her roots in the equine world, a bit of her history in bondage, and her dreams of being a pony as often as practically possible. By the time we parted company that evening, we had a plan for training and a location arranged. And I had a vision for what she would look like tacked up in black and red.

Her first training experience was the usual halting, stumbling, unsettled time most have, but Lyndsey learned quickly and worked hard. After the first session, I gave her assignments to be done daily until we could meet again. She needed some muscle development so she could high step sharply. Lyndsey practiced faithfully and when we met the second time, she was much surer of her steps and far more responsive.

Over several meetings, her training progressed through high steps, to basic gaits, and then crisper and crisper responsiveness to the reins. Verbal commands ceased in time, as they were no longer necessary. I discovered that Lyndsey gains some of her pony headspace from "getting dressed": the more tack she dons, the more pony there seems to be.

We continued to exercise and train regularly in the spring and summer of 2007. In July we worked hard on her tack collection: body suits, boots and decorations. We borrowed horn-hooves, and made a second, shorter tail, for four-legged riding. We were given a saddle. Currently we are working on completing a tack set suitable for four-legged riding.

In August 2007, Kirby, Lyndsey and I went to FetishCon in Tampa. We presented a class on pony play. More than the usual introductory material was covered because we had photographers and producers in the audience. The FetishCon staff set aside a huge play area for us! We gave free cart rides to anyone who wanted one. Keith Humphreys, PonyOATS's official photographer, took dozens of pictures. I had a grand time showing off my ponies!

Chapter Seven
The Inspiration – The Horse

When mankind partnered with equines, civilization changed drastically.

The horse evolved from food animal to companion over the last six thousand years. The value of the horse as a tool has brought humans and equines into an intimate relationship that engenders mutual love and respect. More than a simple catalyst, the horse has proved to be a partner and an influence. Rumor has it that Aristotle liked to be ridden as a pony.

The horse has also become an ever-evolving symbol of wealth and power; in the tribal context, horse ownership conferred status on the owner similar to the standing achieved by modern day racehorse breeders. Even after the horse became a companion and a pastime rather than a working tool, humans continued to classify their inanimate tools in reference to horses: the work capacity of machinery is still measured in horsepower.

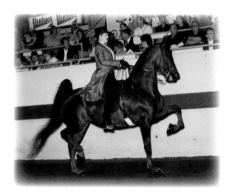

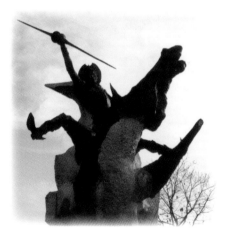

In work, recreation and art, the human and the equine are inseparable.

Top: "Carrie showing Lady Zachary," photographed by Jamie Donaldson, © Jamie Donaldson
Bottom: Don Quixote statue by Teno Aurello.

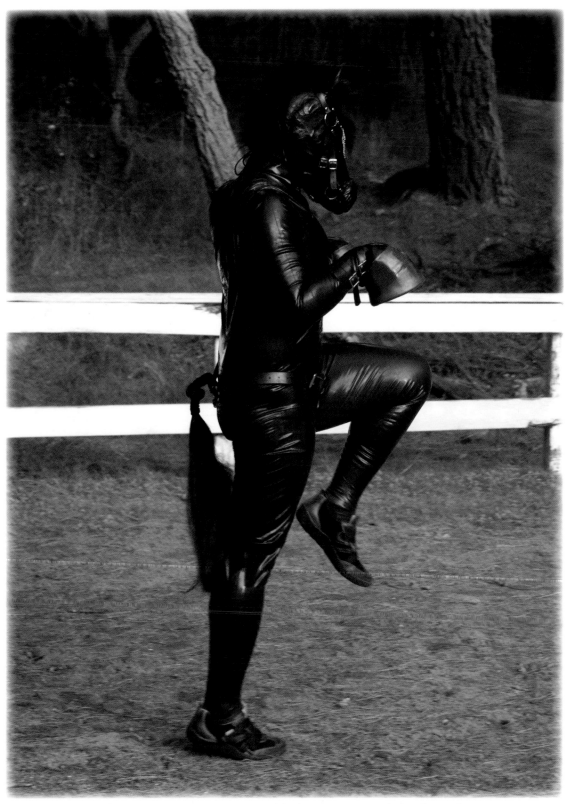

Pony play contains all the possibilities of the human-equine relationship and more.

The horse's influence exceeds mere day to day life. Horses have inspired people to greatness as well as helping them to succeed at greatness. Homer writes of inspired horses charging into battle in the Iliad, virtually with a will of their own. Statuary both ancient and modern shows honored and respected figures of history and literature sitting upon a noble steed. Modern artists use horses to convey a simpler time, connected to the earth, or in abstract juxtapositions of modern life and domestic animal.

The horse has adapted to every need of civilization, even self-actualization. Horses have assisted in helping people achieve all of Maslow's Hierarchy of Needs. The sheer variety of areas where the horse has become invaluable declares the passion people have for this animal.

Pony play contains all these possibilities and more, as players create their own meaning and expression. Horses have participated in human civilization as transportation, food, a hunting and war tool, beast of burden, status symbol, friend, pet, hobby, entertainment, income source and so on. Equestrian activities include racing, farming, ranching, breeding, rodeo, gymkhana, hunting, jumping, cross-country eventing, dressage, equitation, vaulting, rosenback riding, circus performance, war, cart and wagon pulling, logging, pleasure riding, trail riding, endurance riding, herding, aesthetics, polo, theater productions – even babysitting. Each activity has a variety of styles, philosophies and traditions, all of which offer inspiration for pony players

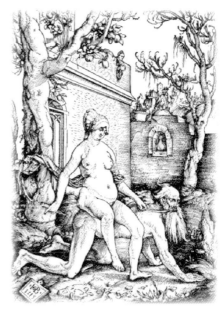

Rumor has it that Aristotle liked to be ridden as a pony.

"Phyllis Riding Aristotle," 1620 woodcut by Hans Bedlung Grien.

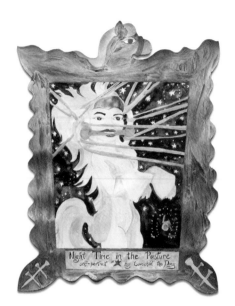

Human ponies capture and embody the spirit of the horse.

Notwithstanding, biological horses possess individual personalities and functions, as do human ponies. Those who are unappreciative of anthropomorphism may not understand the pony player's drive to manifest that passion. Innumerable lovers of horses attribute human characteristics to horses in general, but even more specifically to horses they know personally. Horses exhibit many of the same behavioral characteristics as humans, such as willingness, laziness, excitability, grumpiness, violence, sweetness, gentleness, and downright bitchiness. They do silly things just for their amusement, often out of boredom (and that sometimes amuses the observers as well!). Other attitudes include pride, exhibitionism, psychosis and fear. Each animal expresses a different attitude and response to interactions with people. Regardless of the motivation, the desire to demonstrate abilities reigns strong. Again, the number of examples demonstrates the breadth of interpretation available to players.

Though personalities manifest with different flavors, two main themes prevail regarding human pony attitudes: willingness and willfulness. Most ponies want to be useful, used and needed. Some like to resist. All tend to desire and respect a relationship with their human, much as a biological equine would.

Interacting with biological horses makes plain the interest in pony play. They possess a kinship with humans unlike any other domestic animal. Human ponies capture and embody the spirit of the horse.

Illustration: "Nightmare in the Pasture," Dorian Katz

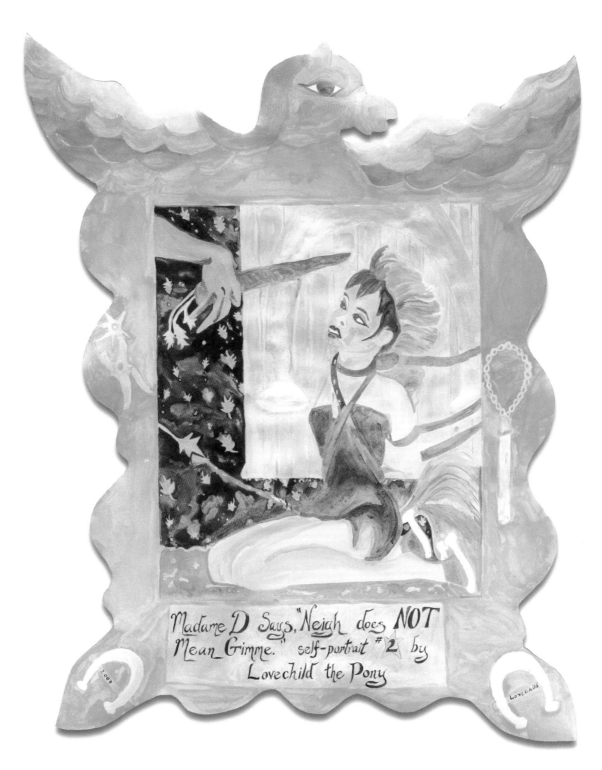

The freedom and joy of pony play has inspired many artists.

Illustration: "Neigh Does NOT Mean Gimme," Dorian Katz

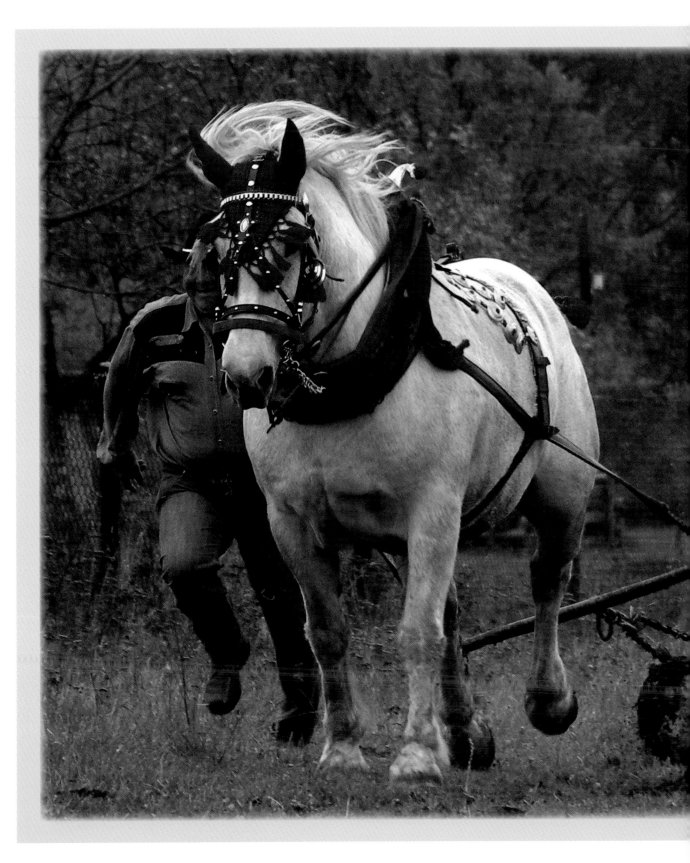

Large photo: © Paulina Dudik, photographer.
Inset photo: © Matthias Kohl. Pupett is a registered trademark of Matthias Kohl.

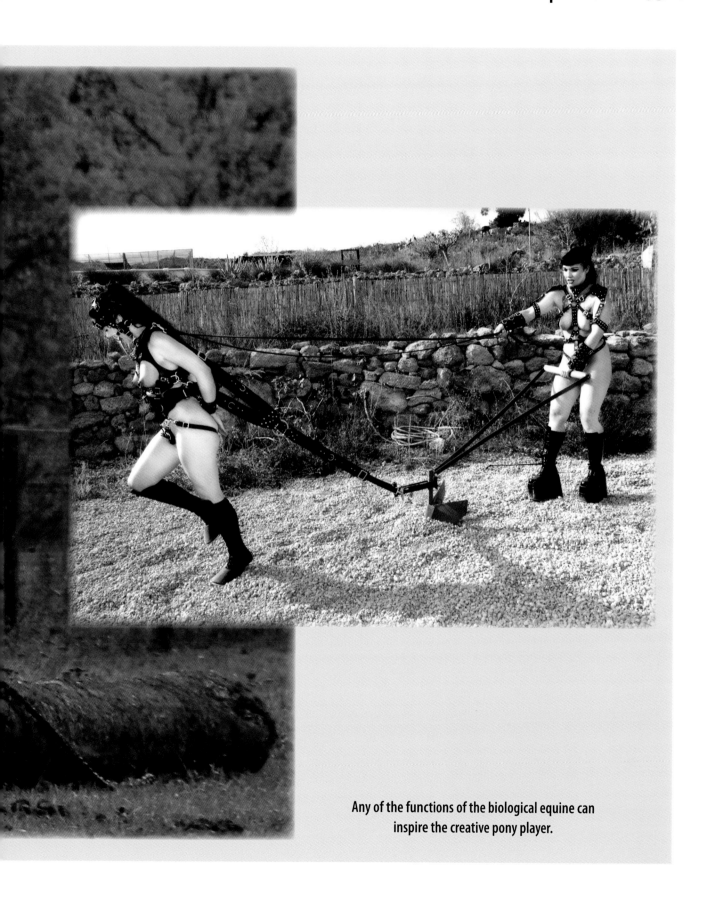

Any of the functions of the biological equine can
inspire the creative pony player.

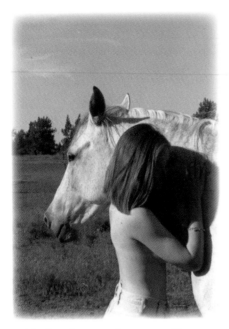

The love between human and horse.

Pegasus Parachute, my mustang mare adopted off the Bureau of Land Management range at six months old, continues to entertain girls in love with horses as she has all her life. From the moment she entered captivity she had a strong will and interesting, even baffling, personality. Not having many options for a herd, she adopted a cat as her companion. She followed the cat around as a filly. As she grew up the cat slept on her rump. In the winter her daily amusement began with a full-out charge around the paddock to culminate in sliding on her side - repeatedly - until she couldn't stand any more. Starting at one end of the paddock she'd run as fast as she could and throw herself down and slide, only to get up and do it again and again until she'd lie still on the ground, barrel and chest heaving from the exertion. No doubt this activity exhausted her angst and need for exercise.

She didn't behave as other horses do. Carrots were beneath her, but offer her dried pineapple and you could get anything out of her. She was sometimes on the bitchy side, but the only thing she really hated was cows. She chased cows incessantly when turned out with them. On one occasion she grabbed hold of a calf by the scruff of the neck with her teeth and shook it as hard as she could – an incident that unfortunately required reimbursing the rancher for damage to his stock. Needless to say, she could not be trusted with them and lost the privilege.

We spent many wonderful hours together as companions, often on the trail. She knew the powers of negotiation. In spite of not having verbal skills, there was no doubt about her desires. At times on the trail she would turn opposite of the rein cue or lean her body away to let me know she preferred another direction. Perhaps she'd try two or three times, sometimes with a struggle; but she'd submit eventually. Sometimes I'd try her route. She tried hard, but still knew her limits. She trained until she sweated and shook and then stopped: enough was enough. She loved adventures. We rode cross-country; she with a gaiety in her step and ears pricked forward, and me two-point in the saddle, exploring for hours at a time. She presented a wonderful example of individualism in all beings.

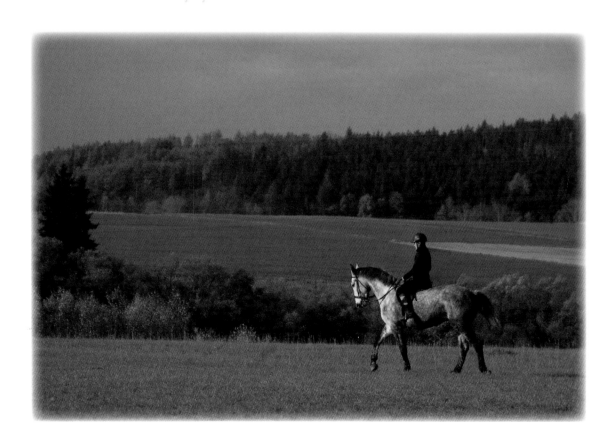

© Paulina Dudik, photographer

Focus: JG-Leathers and "The Creature"

Pony people constantly inspire my imagination with their vision and drive, and none more than JG-Leathers. His integration of other BDSM and fetish interests into his pony play evolved into an extraordinary, pony-inspired sensory device known as "The Creature." Here is his story in his own words, drawings and photographs:

A look back through illustrations that have been preserved from as far back as the pharaohs show that "horse women" (and men) have been around for millennia.

The first appearance of the modern ponygirl took place in the late 1700s, when the printing press made artwork more available to the world. More and more illustrations have slowly surfaced of people engaging in what could be described as pony play. More recently, back in the mid-1950s, drawings and photographs became available for public consumption when John Willie's and Stanton's illustrations and stories became popular, but they were suppressed as much as the authorities of the day could manage.

Now, in the early 21st century, there seems to be a flood of images and videos, and there's even a scene-specific magazine, Equus Eroticus, *devoted to this part of the kink spectrum.*

Until the mid-1980s no one had ever attempted to make any sort of movie or video about horse women or pony girls... and that's where I came on the scene. Jim Rogers and Barbara Behr of House Of Milan were kind enough to do an eight-page photo-spread of my harness designs in Hogtie Magazine *somewhere back around 1982, and at that time we discussed the possibility of doing a video. That came to pass some two years later when I was invited to Los Angeles to supply my harnesses as props for the video. As it turned out, a suitable male lead was not availble, particularly one with the knowledge I had of how the harnesses were to be fitted to the beautiful ladies chosen for the parts of horse women. I ended up being cast as the bad-ass*

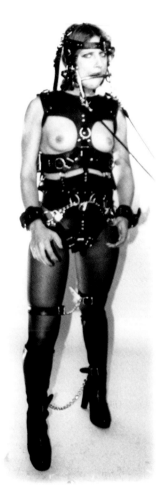

One of the first pre-Creature iterations.

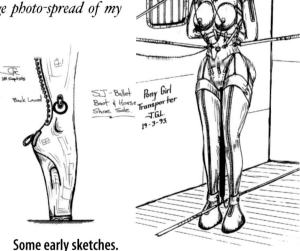

Some early sketches.

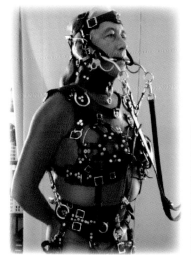 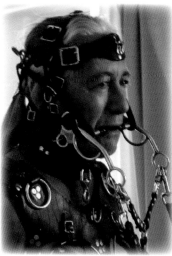 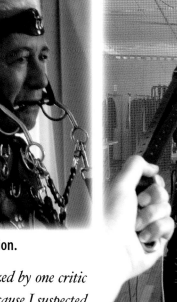

JG-Leathers modeling his own creation.

ranch ramrod "Jay," and was characterized by one critic as a "skinny dickweed." I had to laugh, because I suspected the SOB was just jealous that he couldn't do what I'd gotten to do. The video sold widely and well, both in North America and Europe, and remains a classic of the genre to this day.

Becoming a "human animal" is a fantasy for many. For me, at least, it has to do with depersonalization and objectification. When one is an animal, responsibility departs, and the person who becomes the horse, puppy, cow, or whatever can allow their baser instincts free play. Popular para-psychology? Perhaps so, but I have been fortunate to see many such transformations over the years and greatly admire those who can muster the courage within themselves to go this route.

I have personally been there as well: I designed my own harnesses, bridle and restraint systems. I know them to be both extremely limiting and delightfully controlling in the hands of a skilled Mistress, because I built them to be that way.

Over the past twenty-five years, I've done many presentations about the Human Equine, all with ladies who were willingly bridled, bitted and harnessed. It has always been a delightful experience, and an honor granted by them to me, to control their reins and thus to control them. I thought at first that I was the only one with this particular interest, but obviously I was wrong. Now, Human Equine Groups, web sites, photographs and more videos have turned into a flood tide that is still hard for me to believe.

Truly, pony play is a sensory, sensually and physically rewarding scene, for surrendering freedom and control is a release that only those of us who love it can truly understand. – JG-Leathers, April, 2008

More information and pictures are available on JG-Leathers' website at *www.jg-leathers.com.*

All illustrations and photos have been graciously provided by my friend JG-Leathers, one of the originators of the modern-day pony girl and horse woman scene.

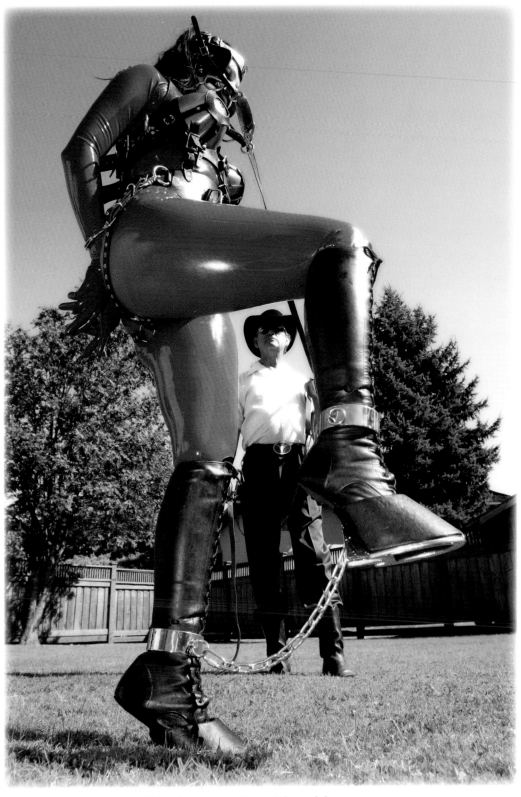

JG-Leathers putting Pupett through her paces.

Chapter Eight
Event Planning: Do It Yourself

T here are only two ways to get what you want: either ask for it from someone who can do it, or *do it yourself*. The latter helps ensure that the end result actually comes together in a way that satisfies your vision.

Assuming that your vision includes developing pony play opportunities in a local community, the first consideration is the time and money required to do so. It takes devotion and commitment to the vision and the communities, especially since the planners rarely fully enjoy the event itself. However, "event oversight" is better than "no event at all." Only the planner decides what returns make it worthwhile.

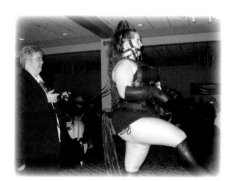

Mystic Storm and Luna, International Pony and Trainer 2008.

Remember, hosting an event means all the responsibility as well as all the blame rests on the planner. The type of event often determines its worth to the individual. Some pony play communities run events as a club which divides the responsibility and work. Nevertheless, someone has to start the process and nurture it.

The next consideration concerns the type of event the community will support. If an ac-

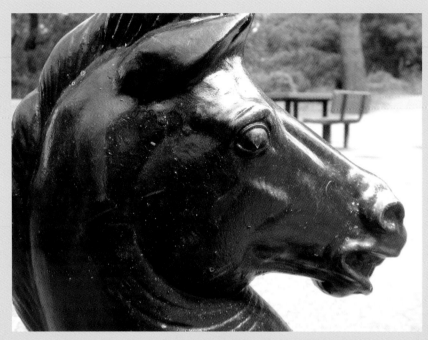

Golden Gate Park location for Picnics in the Park, led by Tipsy.

My Lesson

When I moved to San Francisco, I hit the ground running by attending kinky events immediately. Within two days, just after I got my clothes organized, the SF Pony Munch called to me, and now calls me every month. There, animal role-players enjoy lively conversation and event scheming. The first lesson drilled into me was "Do It Yourself" – from "Mr. Stampede" or Davor, also known as Tipsy pony. His tale of how the San Francisco Pony Munch came into being and evolved into the ongoing official Stampede Munch exemplifies his belief in DIY.

The munch started because he wanted a local social center instead of traveling to San Jose to attend the original Stampede Munch. One thing led to another, and, on the advice of another player, the munch evolved into a consistent watering hole for pony players and those who love them.

That fateful night of my first visit gave me two opportunities. First, my question regarding how to find pony play options in the Bay Area received the answer, "What do you want to do?"

I thought, "Huh, what do I want to do?" My desires had driven me to countless workshops to fill my cup, and now, for the first time, I contemplated the idea of what I wanted to create for the community.

The second offering of the evening presented me with a lead on a private property offered for pony play. Serendipity allowed that I had a car and time for reconnaissance. My doings quickly blossomed into the Pony Play Day events and eventually to the fox hunts at The Ranch.

Photographer: Rebecca Wilcox

tive community of pony players exists, half the work is done. If not, marketing the event locally, nationally or even internationally emerges as the next consideration. The Internet offers a good network base of pony players as well as information on pony play. Research previous regional events, both successful and unsuccessful, to determine how to proceed. Play tends to stay within its own region for the most part, though a few ponies travel. You might wish to poll the greater community to find out what motivates players to schedule time and budget money for travel to a pony event.

Regular activities happen in the San Francisco Bay Area and surrounding communities. There are weekend intensives, such as the Annual Dog and Pony Show in April, Sunday afternoon picnics in Golden Gate Park, and camping events like the fox hunts at The Ranch. Other events, like the Pet Parade in San Jose and the Pony Play Days, also take place all over the SF Bay Area.

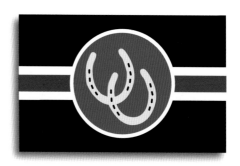

The Pony Pride Flag's creator, Carrie (Mystic Storm), notes, "I hope that this symbol will be carried proudly by ponies everywhere for a very long time to come."

The Fox Hunt

The human fox hunt succeeded in bringing together a diverse group of people in the Bay Area community, including puppy players, pony players, LGBT and heterosexuals, and furries. During the first Pony Play Day, a random group of animal role-play players discussed community building. They wanted to create an all-inclusive event for animal role-players. The magical moment of everyone thinking the same thought in the same moment – *fox hunt* – beautifully exemplifies the cohesiveness of the community's choice. From that point, the fox hunt was destined to come into being.

The first hunt was a lot like hide and seek with teams. Ponies and puppies discovered treats left as a trail that the fox dropped. Another time the fox dropped paper cutouts of fox prints that players picked up along the way. However, the carefully planned BDSM scene that was to be topped by the winning team turned out to be a mob scene that included all the teams in the end. Luckily everyone, including the fox, had an outstanding time anyway. The next hunt ran with one group, comparable to a traditional fox hunt.

Acquiring an appropriate field starts the process of organizing a hunt. A Hunt Master or Mistress officiates the Hunt. Various roles and traditions from traditional fox hunts translate easily to a human fox hunt. The size of the field may limit the numbers of ponies, puppies and trainers that can participate at one time. A small field merely runs heats or separate hunts. Multiple foxes allow for the hunting to continue as long as energy holds out. The hunts run about

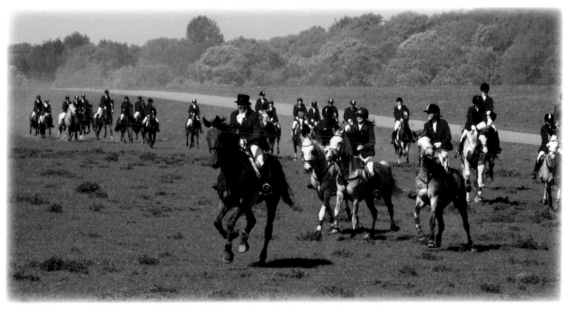

A classic bio-equine fox hunt, our inspiration.

sixty to ninety minutes. Generally it takes multiple hunts to satisfy both the players and foxes. Eventually everyone tires. The hunt boundaries necessitate a visual reminder. Familiarize everyone with the markings. Depending on the size of the field, a field tent with water and first aid supplies may be advisable.

On the day of the event a field secretary organizes the fee, signing of releases, and role sign-up. A check-in time prior to the actual start time helps to get the hunt off on schedule. Organizing teams, not to mention reviewing the rules and parameters of the hunt, takes a while to set up.

The players enjoy seeing the fox head out in anticipation of hunting the quarry. A lead time of twenty to thirty minutes allows the fox time to lay a trail and hide. Assigning a "whipper-in" or two keeps the dogs on the right trail, assisting in control of the hunt in the case of a large field.

One important element to prepare for involves the capture of the fox. Guard against mob mentality, or recruit a tolerant fox. An objective participant, not one of the hunters, such as the Hunt Master or a Fox Monitor, needs to be charged with the fox's safety. Negotiation regarding the capture of the fox takes place before the hunt begins so that the parameters can be communicated to the hunters before they hit the field.

Since the community of this particular group consists primarily of BDSM players, they naturally made a blood sport of the hunt. Fox hunts originally sported in this manner, and the adaptation was rather apropos. The first fox happened to wear a rubber fox suit that he permitted the hunters to cut off in symbolic representation of the dismemberment of the fox from the original

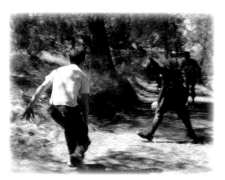

On the chase: Bryan "SMASH" Manternach, the fox, being chased by two puppies.

SAFETY AND ETIQUETTE REGULATIONS FOR THE HUNT

Everyone must check in with the Field Secretary and sign a release *prior to* entering field. Each participant will be asked to select a role in the hunt, as well as read The Ranch disclaimer and rules. This includes spectators.

Allow at least thirty minutes before the scheduled departure of the hunt to have sufficient time to secure equipment and present yourself to the Master/Mistress of the Hunt. Foxhunting is a picturesque sport: A well turned-out hunt participant is a compliment to yourself and the hunt.

Prior to the hunt, participants may be offered a "stirrup cup." This tradition dates back hundreds of years, when the hunt servants would offer a cup of wine or juice prior to the hunt. The Hunt usually meets in the early morning, but a *small* splash of spirits is all part of the tradition.

The Field Master or Mistress leads the hunt at all times. Any questions need to be directed to the Field Master or Mistress during the hunt.

Members with colors displayed on their person have earned the privilege to ride directly

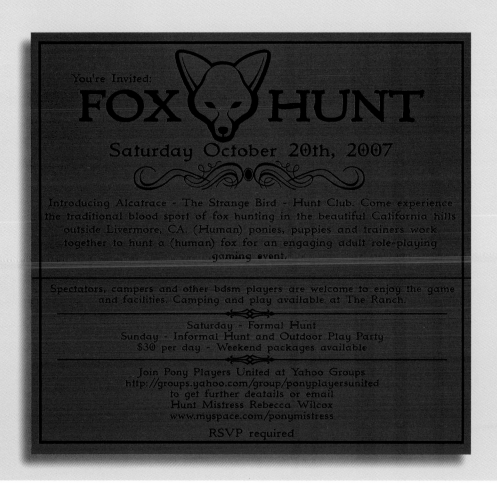

behind the Field Master/Mistress. Tradition mandates the following order within the field: FIRST FIELD; Field Master/Mistress, Sr. Members with Colors, Jr. Members with Colors, Sr. Members without Colors, Juniors, Guests. SECOND FIELD; Hill Top Master, Members with Colors, Guests. The Staff always has the right of way, as do the hounds. Senior members my invite others to pass them.

Colors are earned by the member and awarded by the Hunt Master/Mistress.

Please stay within the boundary markers during the hunt.

No smoking on the field.

Attend to your own safety at all times.

(regional concern) Watch your step at all times. *Beware* of rattlesnakes. If you see a rattlesnake, STOP, especially if it is coiled, and yell, "Rattlesnake."

Announce hazards to the hunt member behind you in a voice only loud enough for that person to hear you. Please do not yell. "Ware hole," "Ware wire," etc., is proper.

The hunt staff and the hounds have the right of way on all trails, roads, etc.

"Coffee-housing," or chatting, is undesirable in the hunt field.

If you are fortunate enough to view the quarry and the hounds are hunting the line, *keep still and quiet* until they have passed, then face the direction the game has taken and point your hat or whip in the direction he has taken.

Report property damages to the Field Master, who reports to the Master/Mistress of the Hunt.

Leave no trace.

Ponies and Riders must stay connected by a lead line or reins at all times.

Hounds must be under verbal control of the Master/Mistress of the hounds at all times.

Unless safety demands, animals are requested not to use verbal communication.

Capture of the fox requires at least four hunt participants, including one pony and rider, and the Huntsman [Master/Mistress of the Hounds].

The hounds my hold the fox at bay until the required participants arrive to capture him.

The punishment of the fox may not commence until the designated Fox Monitor is present.

When the Fox is captured, the Hunt Master/Mistress or designated Fox Monitor oversees the safety of the fox as well as ensuring that hunters adhere to the negotiated parameters.

A Hunt Potluck follows the hunt in the tradition of the "hunt breakfast." Following the meet, everyone enjoys a picnic meal. Please bring a lunch and/or something to share.

tradition. The sport of the capture may also include whipping, flogging, violation, knife play, caning and the like. Restraining and caging often prolong the play with the fox. Sometimes the play continues on into the night. However, the fox receives rest breaks, food, water and occasionally massage. He's a renewable resource.

Helpful fox hunt terminology

Cover – Any area where the fox may take shelter, usually a wood or thicket.

Dealt With – Euphemism for killing the fox (also known as accounted for, dispatched, punished, et al).

Draw – Encouraging the hounds into a cover in search of the fox.

Draw a blank – To draw a cover without finding a fox.

Field Master/Mistress – The leader of the hunt.

Fox Monitor – Person charged with the safety of the fox.

Given Best – When the fox is allowed to escape to be hunted another day.

Hunt Master/Mistress – Person responsible to organize and control the hunt.

Huntsman or Master/Mistress of the Hounds – Person in charge of the hounds, This person carries the horn and directs the hounds with the use of her voice and the use of the horn itself.

Line – The route taken by the fox.

Meet – Where the hunters meet before the hunt.

Own – Hounds are said to own the line when they pick up the trail.

Point Rider – A Whipper-In or member of the field positioned at a strategic point on the edge of a cover to alert the Huntsman if the quarry breaks.

Staff – The Huntsman or Master/Mistress of the Hounds, Fox Monitor and Whipper-Ins.

Riot – When the hounds chase after other animals rather than the fox.

Tally Ho – The fox has been sighted.

Tally Ho Away – The fox has left cover.

Tally Ho Back – The fox has returned to cover.

Tally Ho Over – The fox has changed paths.

Voice – Sound made by the hounds when they are on the trail. (Also known as speak, giving tongue, giving voice, being in cry, etc.

Ware – A call to signal obstacle or reprimand, e.g., "Ware Riot!", "Ware Hole!", "Ware Wire!", Ware Rock!", "Ware Rattlesnake!"

Whippers-In – The people assigned by the Huntsman, usually in Senior colors, to ride out to the sides of the hounds and keep them within the property boundaries. Their main job is to keep the pack together and prevent the hounds from "running riot." To help them control the pack they carry hunting whips. They are also called upon to signal the view of the fox by yelling "tally ho."

View halloe (pronounced, view hello) – When "Tally Ho" is called.

Each hunt adds more elements of a traditional hunt. Built on a long-standing, rich tradition, human fox hunts have the advantage of translating that tradition into play.

Pony Show

Many ponies, especially the highly competitive and exhibitionist types, request a pony show. Unfortunately, people can sometimes get wrapped up in their egos. Biological equines don't care if they get a ribbon or not – usually they hate having it flapping in their face. They do care about pleasing the rider/driver/handler. The Dog and Pony Show was forced to curtail competitions when hurt feelings and negative competitiveness ruined the events.

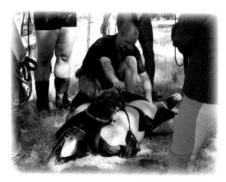

Good puppy! Spike, a German Shepherd pup, skinning a rubber fox.

However, human pony play competitions can offer an excellent opportunity to exhibit the ponies and their training if the competition supports the positive aspects of competition and creates a safe environment for all. Putting on a pony show requires attending to many details, including, but not limited to: finding a space, a judge, prizes, a way to get the information out, and all the fees, permits, insurance and safety precautions to go with it.

Competitions and workshops often go well hand in hand. Deliberating with other players and consulting other planners who have executed such events can help. A few elements to ponder include: the number of expected entries, the space necessary for the entries and spectators, the judge(s), how to best support the players as well as the greater community, the impact on the site and innocent bystanders, what kind of classes to offer and positive marketing. Mutual respect between ponies and judge(s) may make or break the competition. Find a judge who is likely to inspire the players' respect. The judge needs to know pony play, the rules of the classes, and how to evaluate objectively. It helps if the awarding of the prizes affirms and supports peace and proves justifiable. Although judging involves subjectivity, it truly involves more than a mere opinion. Workshops build the community as well as helping people know where to start in their play. Community building holds many rewards worth the demands.

Pony play competitions can be found around the United States; most are posted to various pony interest groups and websites. Many people have found ways to make these events happen. One DIY-er designed the Pony Pride flag in support of the greater pony community.

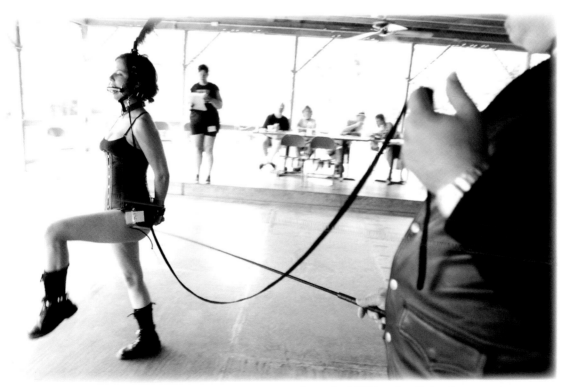

Ponygirl Cymbra, "Sexiest Pony" winner from the 2005 Leather Retreat.

Possible Classes and Descriptions

In Hand – Trainer and pony demonstrate overall ability to work together as well as show their look. Class judged on demonstration of clear communication; performance of in-hand techniques which may include walk, trot, stand, back; one minute of creative expression; and overall presentation.

Costume – Class judged on creativity of pony and trainer/handler expression. Ponies may enter alone or in pairs; however, overall look with a handler improves score.

Equitation – Rider's ability to communicate with the horse.

Over-fences classes – Horse's movement, manners, way of going, and jumping form, over a course of jumps.

Pleasure classes – Unlike the flat and over-fences classes, the horse's movement is not as important as its manners, temperament, and suitability for the rider.

Agility – Obstacle course event: Event scored and timed. Points deducted for touching or avoiding obstacles. [Optional: Blindfold]

Work/Draft – The endurance test proves ability to move weight, judged by time and distance.

Cart – Trainer and pony demonstrate ability to work the cart. Class judged on both the demonstration of the ability of pony and trainer to work together and athletic ability of the pony.

Cart Racing – Timed event.

Classes may be further divided by the horse or rider's experience or the height, type, or breed of the pony.

Best of Show – The sum total of scores for events entered over the course of the show calculates overall score for Best of Show. Ties determined by in-hand competition determined by the judge.

1st – 5 points; 2nd – 4 points; 3rd – 3 points; 4th – 2 points; 5th – 1 point

Class options: Gymkhana-type classes such as Barrel Racing, Egg Toss, Dollar Bill and Pole Bending; English based events such as Stadium Jumping, Cross Country Eventing and Dressage; or Rodeo events like Bronco Riding, Timed Sheep Tie and Best Cow Horse (even more fun with human bovines).

Ideas for "everyone wins" type of events: Best Whinny, Best Trick, Best Coordinated Costume, Most Original Costume, Sexiest Pony... be creative!

See class descriptions from biological equine shows.

Participants may be excused from the ring for any behavior that puts the pony or other exhibitors at risk, or for any rude, disruptive or dangerous behavior by the pony or trainer.

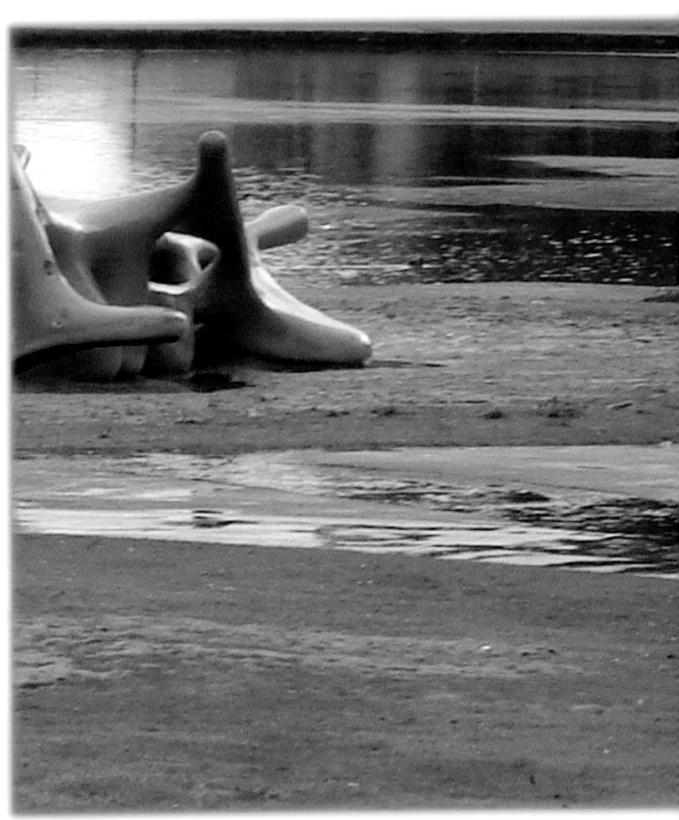

Pony Play Day at Lake

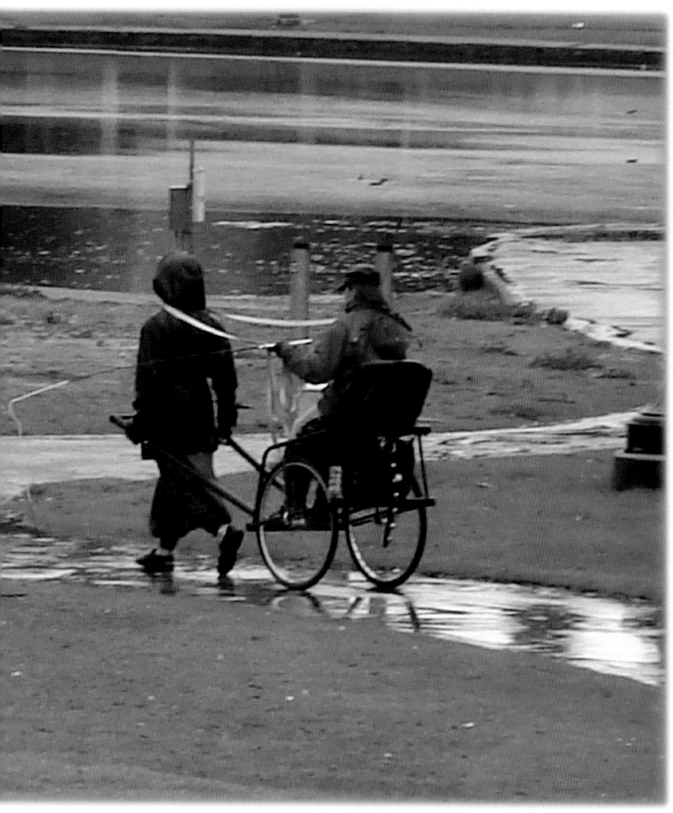

Merritt, Oakland, CA 2006.

I enjoy training ponies. I hope my ponies enjoy being trained. We believe this game, if played for real, is for freely consenting adult volunteers only, and forcing someone into it by any sort of coercion, no matter how subtle, will not help.

One particular pony I played with had been around the scene for a while. When she came over to play, I attached the leading rein to her collar and led her to my tack room to be harnessed up. Once there I put her wrist and ankle cuffs on her appropriate limbs. I put the harness over her shoulders. I clipped the wristlets to ropes from a couple of overhead attachment points, the anklets to points on a board on which she stands. I pulled on and securde the ropes so that she was comfortably but securely spread-eagled. The bridle went on fairly easily, though its complexity was something of a problem over long hair.

All the time I did this I was talking to her, as one would a real pony. I wanted to reassure her as I handled her, made adjustments, and ensured everything was just so. Ponies love such attention. They do like to know that you're taking care, looking after them properly.

Once I had her all harnessed up, I lowered her arms, clipped the wrist cuffs to the waist belt and led my Sweet Lass out for her first pony training session. I had checked to be sure that everything was comfortable, and that nothing pinched or chafed. She was a bit cool from standing immobile for a while, so once I led her out I thought I ought to warm her up.

At first we were walking normally, then high-stepping, then jogging. Every so often, at a random point in the circuit, I would pull the far rein to have her turn and circle in the other direction. At this stage I was still explaining everything to her verbally, as well as with the reins, so that she could begin to get used to the feel.

Once I'd warmed her up on the lunge I took her for a session of "long reining." This means I led her around the garden, walking behind at a reasonable distance, steering her by the reins. Again I spoke the commands as I gave them via the reins, but began tailing this off as she began to get the hang of trusting the reins. I'd lead her towards the trees, leaving the command to the very last moment, randomly turning left or right, or halting her and having her side-step and/or back off. I was checking with a sharp word any tendency to anticipate the command via the reins, and later with the whip if I felt it necessary. The session lasted quite a while, until she was obediently walking exactly as commanded, with no verbal assistance from me.

Then, just to make sure she had fully learned to trust the reins, I took out a blindfold, put it over her eyes, and carried on. Again, I at first reinforced the commands via the reins with spoken commands, but soon let her take all her clues from the reins.

She walked, she pranced, and she trotted at my command and even cantered, though I was a little careful at such an early stage and without the protection of the knee pads.

Anyway all good things must come to an end, especially when something even more interesting is in view, so when I had decided she learned all she needed to know before being put between the shafts, I took her over to the sulky and harnessed her to it.

I led her out by the leading rein from her collar, and took her around the garden a turn or so, to get the feel of the empty sulky. It is not a burden at all, but it does constrain the way you move to an extent and the jingling trace chains and the feel of something following close behind can be unsettling at first; I wanted this pony to take it very gradually.

I left her like that for a little while, and made a bit of a fuss over her by stroking to her and making sure she was happy to go on to the next stage. (Though if she weren't happy she'd have had to do it anyway – that, or end the scene with a safeword – and she knew it!)

I love the view from the seat of a sulky. I love it no matter the pony I have harnessed, but I especially love to see a nice filly. I can't claim this filly is yet ready to race, but she was spirited, game, and pretty in her own way. So, I made myself comfortable, adjusted where I sat so that the cart was nicely balanced with just a few pounds on the waist & just enjoyed the view for a while.

I explained that if I'm enjoying the ride I stroke the pony's back & rump sensuously with my whip as she pulls me along. I did it to demonstrate. She seemed to appreciate this a good deal, judging by the way she moved her hindquarters.

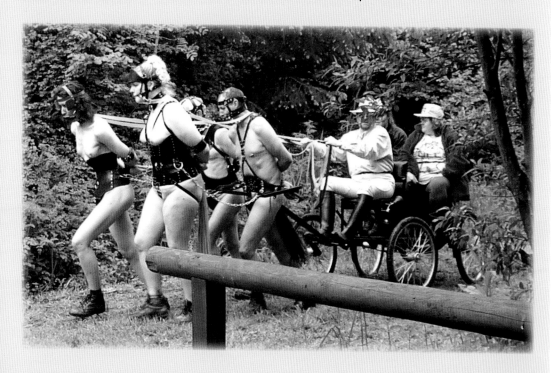

So I then just carried on where the long reining left off. I took her this way and that, in circles, figures of eight, around the trees, up to the trees, turning or halting at the last moment.

Backing up is something ponies find very difficult, as they can't turn their heads to look behind, of course. Anyone who has ever tried to reverse a car with trailer or caravan attached will begin to appreciate the difficulty, not just for the pony, but for the rider too! At such times the whip and reins can seem to get in an awful tangle, especially while you're learning.

It is true, too, that though I can train my ponies as best I can, drivers will generally not accept training in quite the same way. Every driver will use the reins and whip in a slightly different way. The most common fault, particularly by those who have ridden real horses (and especially horses hired from riding schools) is to pull too hard on the reins. A horse has a much harder mouth than does a human, and is much stronger and has probably been mauled about a lot before. Anyway, human ponies just have to learn the meaning of each individual driver's techniques as best they can, and since the driver has a whip too, they must learn as fast as they can.

I had her pirouette in a side-step, so that I just sat and was spun in the one place without moving. I had her prance and trot to order. Then a turn onto the other diagonal, a brisk double flick with the whip into a canter from a standing start. A turn at the back of the arena to go across the back in a fine, high-stepping walk, across to the middle.

Then a circle around, walking, trotting, prancing and cantering, in ever-decreasing circles until we were pirouetting in the centre of the arena. Then backing off. If the applause were to warrant it, I would have her go down to take a bow with me alongside, then lead her off by the reins.

We practiced this routine a few times, as above and with variations. The great thing about events that they give a point to the routine training that has to be done by a pony and driver before they become really proficient, elegant and precise in the way they work together.

I hope to welcome her back, perhaps for more advanced training someday, even if it is as a driver for some of my other ponies (as she suggested it might be). I'm sure she'd have no shortage of volunteers! I think that this pony was willing enough and enjoyed it rather a lot.

For one of the many things I have learned is that, given a little consideration for the pony it can be just as much fun for the pony as for the driver. When both enjoy it is wonderful!

– Sir Guy, of The Tawsingham Society and The Other Pony Club of Great Britain

Conclusion
End on a Good Note

It's about play, so play to your heart's content.

Passion guides us to do what must be done; when it brings joy and satisfaction, it claims its worth. So many people find worth in pony play when the type of play speaks to them. Story after story after story, far beyond those that make it to the public's ear, tell the tale of inner joy. The pony community continues to grow strong, building within itself the support necessary to provide the space for play in safety and harmony.

Play becomes scene when the players understand the capabilities, boundaries and interests of everyone involved. The mental, emotional and physical baseline changes from play session to play session, just as they do from day to day in life. Trainers and handlers grow in their skills as they learn to adapt and guide their ponies through personal development, physical endurance and technical skill. Ponies facilitate the play through honest response and willingness, even if that means the willingness to resist based on negotiation. Communication and cooperation cultivate each player's needs into beautiful expressions of creativity. The interaction weaves back and forth as the partnership develops, perhaps exploring aspects that never would have evolved without the particulars of pony play. Knowing what each player desires to get out of the play builds a clear path that brings them to a happy end.

In order to keep the play safe, remember each pony responds differently and may respond differently on a new day. Expect the unexpected. Monitor safety issues, especially regarding bondage and training equipment, each time as if it were the first time. Prepare yourself to suspend reality while maintaining safety parameters – multitasking in a big way. The pony focuses so hard on being a pony and listening to the handler that she probably won't think about her needs.

Maintaining a trouble-shooting attitude assists in doing discovery around what motivates the behavior. Ponies act out for a reason; the play evolves through the choices made. May the play be a positive experience for everyone. Above all else – END ON A GOOD NOTE.

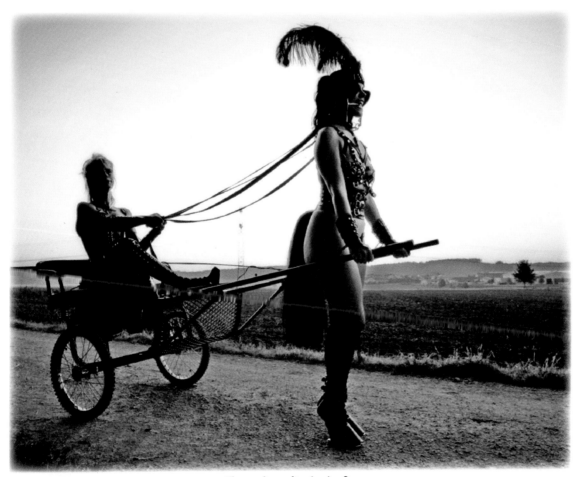

The end... or beginning?

Appendix A
Gaits

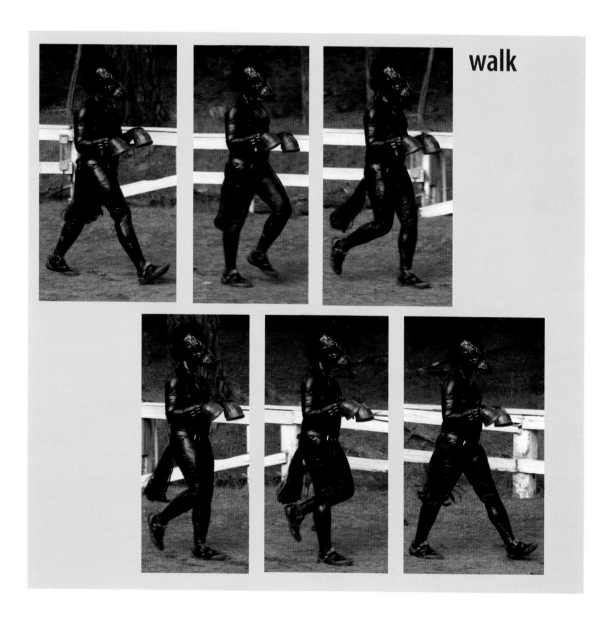

walk

trot

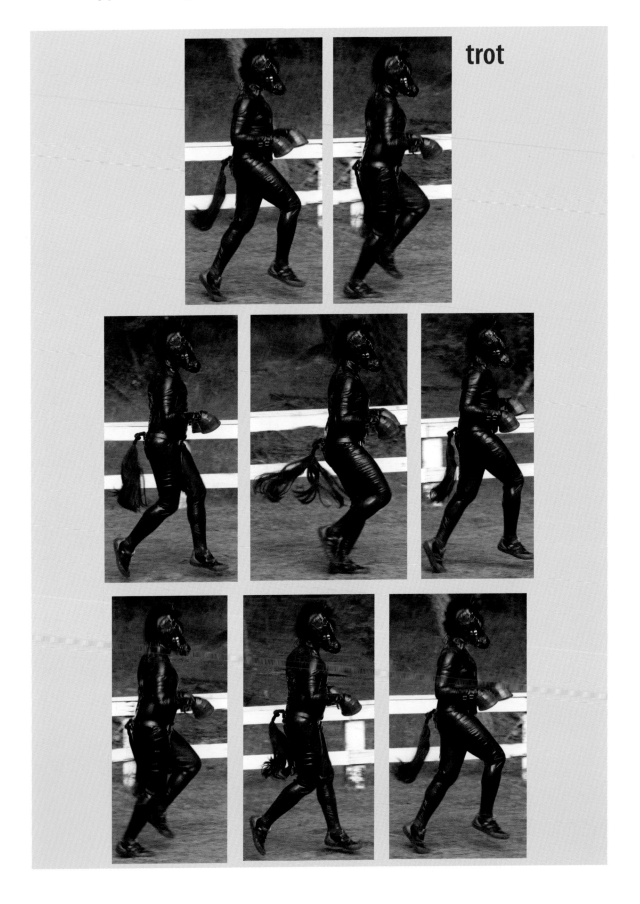

canter

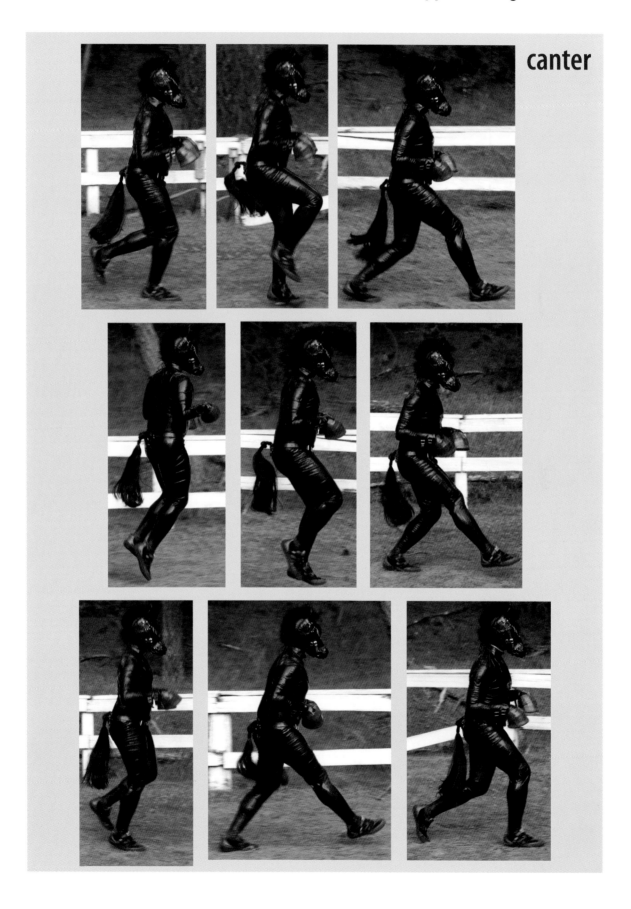

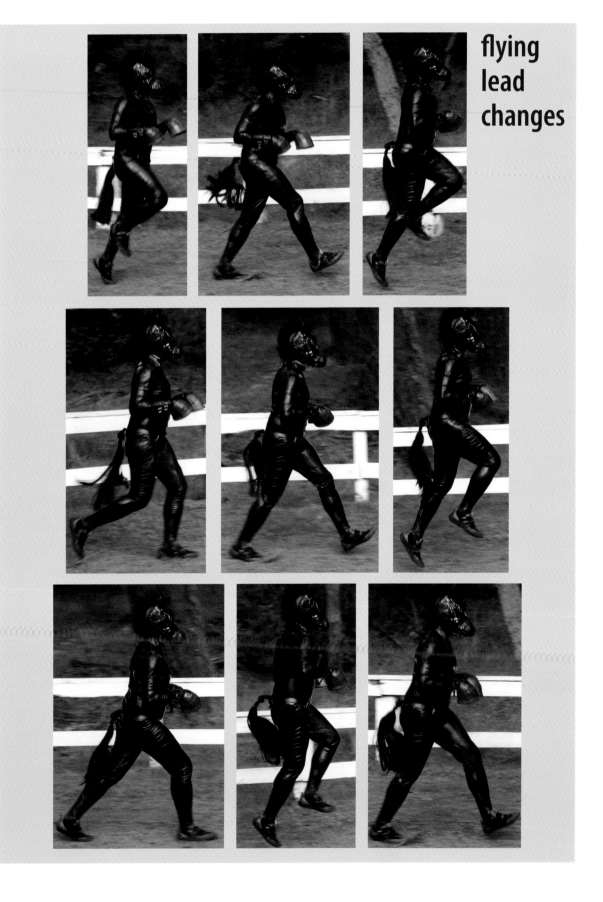

flying
lead
changes

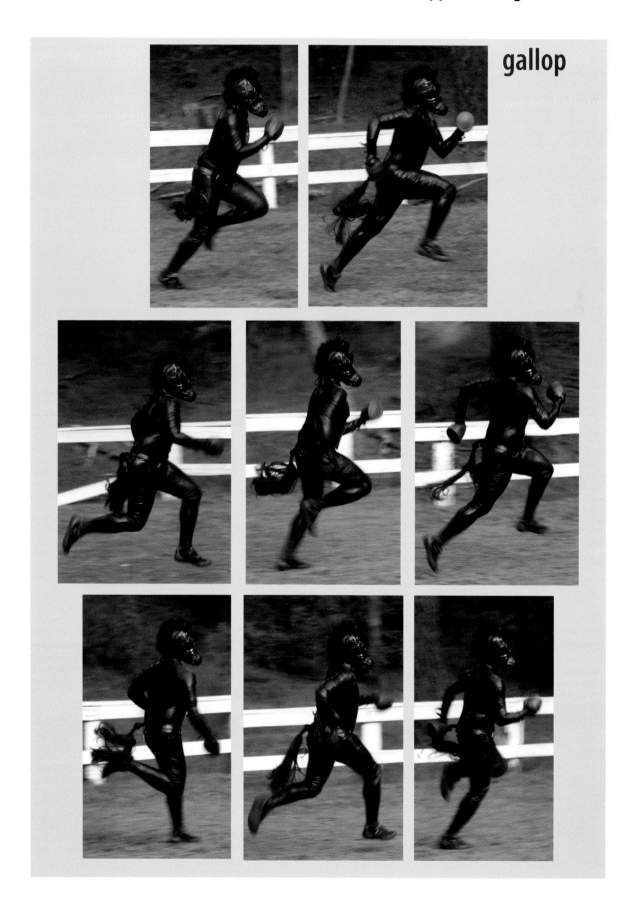

gallop

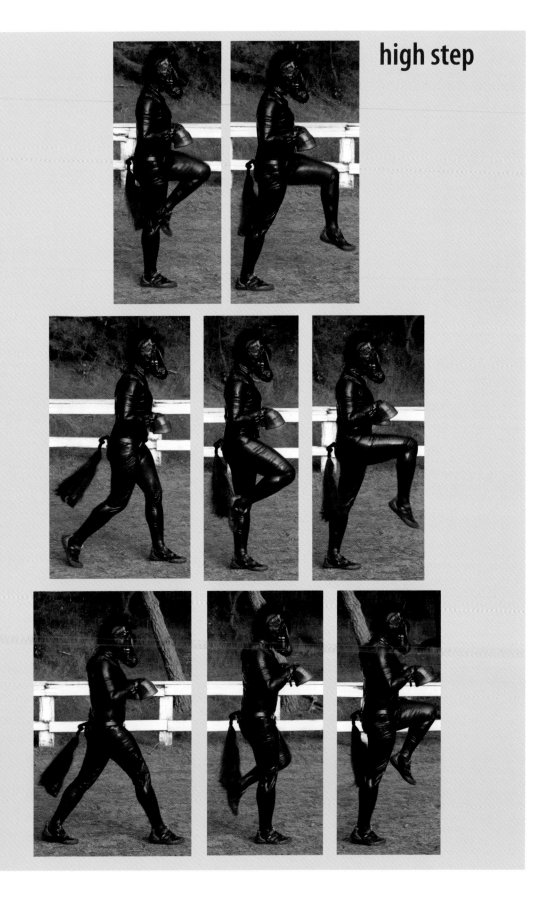

high step

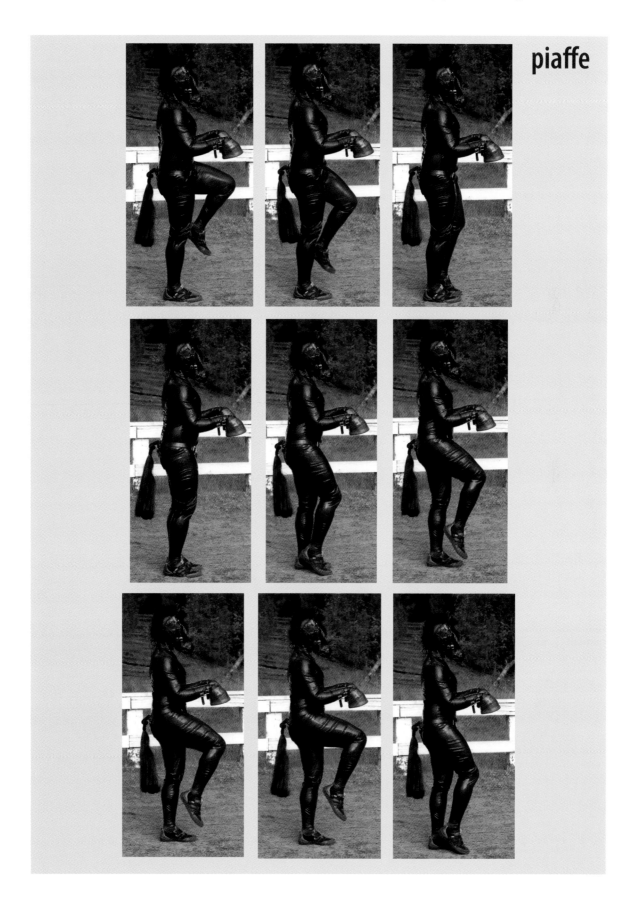

piaffe

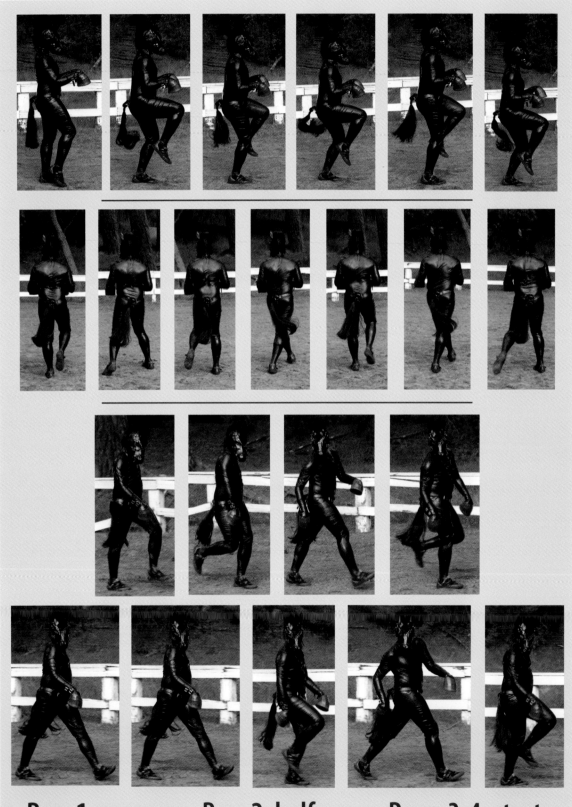

Row 1: passage.   Row 2: half-pass.   Rows 3-4: strut.

Appendix B
Quick Release Knot

The quick release knot allows for a secure tie point with the flexibility to untie in seconds. The knot holds thousands of pounds of pressure without losing integrity of the knot or ability to untie. In the case of biological equines the fence or halter tends will be more likely to break before the rope does. It is reasonably safe as long as some one is within reaching distance. The knot translates well into pony play as well as other purposes. However, you have to beware of cunning ponies who learn to untie the knot for themselves.

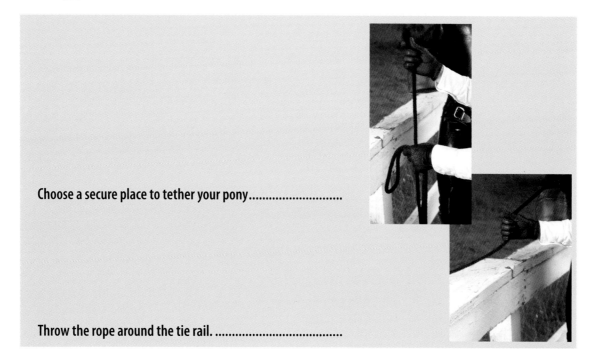

Choose a secure place to tether your pony............................

Throw the rope around the tie rail. ....

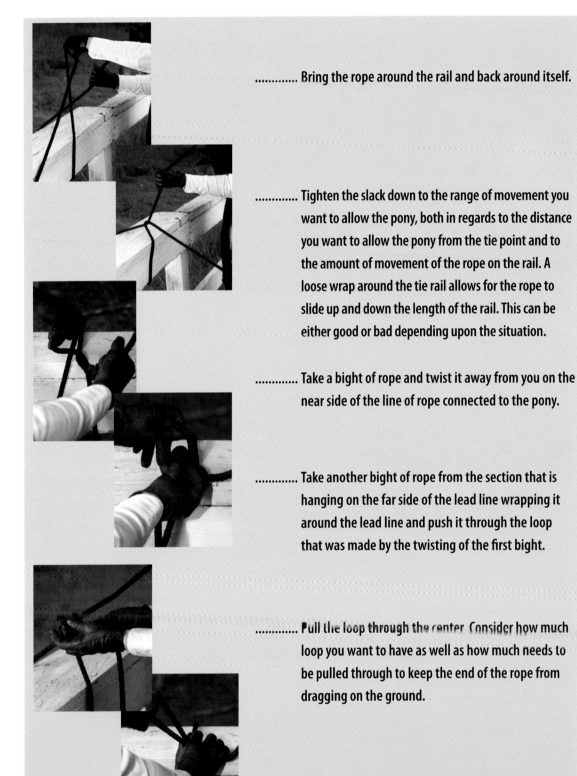

.... Bring the rope around the rail and back around itself.

.... Tighten the slack down to the range of movement you want to allow the pony, both in regards to the distance you want to allow the pony from the tie point and to the amount of movement of the rope on the rail. A loose wrap around the tie rail allows for the rope to slide up and down the length of the rail. This can be either good or bad depending upon the situation.

.... Take a bight of rope and twist it away from you on the near side of the line of rope connected to the pony.

.... Take another bight of rope from the section that is hanging on the far side of the lead line wrapping it around the lead line and push it through the loop that was made by the twisting of the first bight.

.... Pull the loop through the center. Consider how much loop you want to have as well as how much needs to be pulled through to keep the end of the rope from dragging on the ground.

.... Use one hand to pull the knot tight while the other hand holds the position secure.

Finished knot...

You now have a secure tie. ....

To untie, grab the free end with one hand and pull hard. The knot unties in seconds. ....

Appendix C
Pony Play Glossary

Action – frame of movement as the pony moves out.

Aids – signals communicating instructions to the pony.

> Natural aids – hands, body and voice of trainer.

> Training/Artificial aids – equipment used to communicate instructions.

Basic English seat or English Pleasure – umbrella term for riding English style with the characteristic saddle and using direct reining, where the horse is ridden with contact on the rein and guided with pressure on the bit.

BDSM – erotic activities that involve any or all of the following: bondage, discipline, Dominance/submission power exchange, sadism and masochism.

Bit – piece of tack for the mouth that communicates specific messages to the pony dependent upon the function it's designed for. Different bits elicit different responses from the pony.

Bitless bridle – a headstall without a bit.

Boots – leg protection for the pony.

Bottom – person who takes the role of the one being controlled, in this case the pony.

Breast plate – tack item that holds the saddle in place with straps that cross the chest.

Bridle – pony headgear complete with headstall, bit and reins.

Bronc riding – a timed rodeo event where the pony tries to unseat the rider.

Browband – a strap that connects one side of the headstall across the forehead of the pony that helps hold the bridle in place.

Cabriole originally describes a trained movement of the biological equine that involves jumping straight up into the air and kicking the back legs out behind parallel to the ground. In pony play, the pony jumps into the air tucking one leg up and kicking the other leg out behind.

Canter - a controlled, three-beat gait performed by a horse. When performed by a human pony it looks like a child's horse gait or skipping on one side. The leading leg always stays ahead of the following leg. The lead leg is determined by the leg closest to the trainer or inside of the arena or vault. It has two beats with the emphasis on the leading leg: DUH-dum, Duh-dum,...

> **Counter-canter** – deliberately taking the wrong lead.
> **Flying lead change** – changing canter leads in the air without losing the rhythm.
> **Continuous flying lead changes** – looks like skipping.

Carriage pony – a light, elegant pony suitable for show cart or formal carriage work.

Cart pony – heavier, more athletic pony suitable for cart and wagon work.

Cold-blood – generic term for heavy-boned work ponies, usually of a particularly docile temperament.

Collection – the quality of movement by the pony which engages the full musculo-skeletal systems in a manner that produces clear, energized movement within the frame of the pony's natural range of movement. Generally the movement pushes forward into the bit becoming more fully expressed. It presents as perfectly controlled freedom of movement with both impulsion and suspension.

Colt – uncastrated or young male pony.

Cooler – rug, or blanket, to keep the pony from cooling off too quickly after hard **exercise**.

Cue – signal to the pony to perform a specific behavior.

Curb chain – piece of tack that runs from one side of the bit to the other under the pony's chin.

Dominance – exercising control, authority or influence.

Dressage – a specific form of riding that emphasizes the gymnastic athletic abilities of the equine through standardized training methods that maximize all the characteristics of a ideal riding horse. It's often referred to as horse ballet as the participants are graceful and elegant in their movement. Through dressage, a horse demonstrates exceptional athletic ability, willingness to perform, and partnership between equine and rider. At its highest level it appears to be relaxed and effortless.

Engagement – when the pony is correctly on the bit and working toward self carriage.

Extend – the lengthening of the stride within a particular gait, while still maintaining balance and control.

Filly – young female pony.

Full Pass – lateral movement seen in dressage in which the horse moves sideways only.

Gaits – various speeds and rhythms the horse can go.

Gallop – the fastest gait, or running pace. It is faster and covers more ground than the canter.

Gelding – castrated male pony.

Girth – a strap that goes around the pony to hold the saddle on.

Giving Rein – releasing pressure on the bit.

Green – inexperienced pony.

Green broke – when the pony is just learning to accept the bridle, saddle, harness, vehicle, and handling.

Ground work – any training of the pony that occurs with the trainer on the ground.

Half Halt – bringing the pony to higher degree of balance and attention by using aids to check momentum. For example a slight tap of the bit without asking for a "halt."

Half-pass – a lateral movement seen in dressage, in which the horse moves forward and sideways at a diagonal. The legs cross as the pony moves forward, balanced and in rhythm.

Halt – an engaged stop.

Halter or Headcollar – tack item that restrains the head. Used for leading the pony in-hand or tying the pony to a secure point.

Hand – standard of measuring biological equine height, 1 hand equals 4". A pony is measured from the ground to the top of the shoulder. A 5'3" human would typically be about a 15.3 hand pony.

Hand gallop – a controlled gallop used to show a ground-covering stride in competition.

Handler – person who takes on the roll of caretaking of the pony.

Headspace - a variety of mental and emotional conditions that a pony player identifies as the particular frame of reference that he or she operates from while playing. This includes several levels of consciousness defined according to the amount of disengagement from the everyday frame of reference or the intensity of the experience.

Headstall – the main part of the bridle that goes over or around the head that attaches to either side of the bit, holding it on.

Hot-blood – a pure blood or pony of fiery temperament.

Impulsion – light, elastic thrust of the pony's movement. It creates the power of the collected gait necessary to perform highly disciplined movements of the higher levels of disciplined training. Movements such as the passage, piaffe, pirouette, tempi changes, and the collected gaits, as well as the extended gaits, rely on this principle. Impulsion is also associated with the suspension of the trot and canter. The emphasis of the movement is forward.

In-hand – working or handling the pony utilizing ground work. Generally, any handling of the pony involving restraint.

Jog – Western style trot, usually much slower and lower to the ground than an English style trot.

Kink – sexual activity that is outside what is considered sexually normative.

Lateral work – when the pony moves out sideways.

Levade –when a four-legged pony stands up on its rear legs in a controlled manner.

Long reining or ground driving – training the pony with long reins from a greater distance than in hand, usually in preparation to accept riders or to train to cart.

Lope – Western style of canter, usually slower and flatter.

Lunging – training process to teach gaits and voice commands, as well as exercise technique utilizing the circle, or vault.

Mare – older female pony.

Martingale – a piece of tack used to prevent the pony from lifting the head too high.

Maslow's Hierarchy of Needs – physiological, security, love and belonging, esteem, experience purpose, meaning and potential, and self-actualization.

Munch – typically a fetish-based social gathering where like minded folks enjoy casual conversation and food.

Natural gaits– the gaits ponies produce without special training. May be particular to specific ponies.

Neck reining – Western method of turning the pony using pressure on the neck with the reins.

On the bit – when the pony accepts contact with the trainer through slight tension on the bit, yielding to the trainer's will while moving forward with energy.

Passage - a highly elevated, collected and extremely powerful trot that moves with great impulsion. The pony appears to trot in slow motion.

Piaffe - originally used in battle to keep the horse focused, warm, and moving, ready to move forward into battle. The pony collects and trots in place or nearly in place. The center of gravity keeps the pony forward, ready to move. The pony calmly raises each foot with great impulsion without any suspension. The rhythm stays free and light as one foot always remains on the ground. There is a juxtaposition of great energy and control.

Pirouette – technically a turning around on one foot. In human pony play, a pirouette often translates into a circle around the trainer. The pony remains slightly turned toward the direction of travel at any gait. However, a circus pony may perform a pirouette like a dancer.

Play – when people engage in the activity of pony role-play.

Push-button – a pony that does what it's trained to do automatically.

Put through his paces – to take the pony through known training level and/or working of the gaits.

Rack or Racking – in pony play, it is the high step gait sometimes referred to as parade step. It is a highly regimented gait with equal intervals between each step.

Rein – tack item used to communicate signals from the trainer's hands to the bit in the pony's mouth.

Rein back – backing in a straight line on the trainer's command.

Reining - a Western style of pony play where the trainer guides the horses through a precise pattern of circles, spins, and stops at the lope or gallop. It's the Western equivalent of Dressage. The pony and trainer perform a demanding pattern of movement as a team without obvious aids.

Resistance (Play) – when the pony refuses to yield, co-operate or submit to the trainer within a consensual scene context.

Rug – heavy weight blanket.

Run – fastest gait, or gallop.

Running Walk – a walk characterized by greater speed and smoothness.

Saddle – a piece of tack that enables a rider to sit comfortably upon the pony.

Saddle bags – storage pouches attached to the saddle or surcingle.

Saddle pad – blanket or padding used as a cushion between the pony and the saddle.

SM or Sadomasochism – erotic sexual play involving the giving and receiving of pain.

Scene – word used within the BDSM community for a play session between consenting adults. Typically it has a beginning and ending point. It's used here as a word to describe the role-playing session.

Schooling arena – enclosed area for training ponies.

Self carriage – when the pony performs disciplined training exercises without needing the training aids.

Sheet – lightweight cover for keeping the pony clean and warm.

Shy – when a pony moves fearfully away from an object or noise.

Side reins – anchored reins that hold a pony's head in place during lunging.

Simple Change – trotting or walking transition between one lead at the canter to the other lead.

Spanish walk – specially trained walk with a full extension of the legs reaching forward and nearly parallel to the ground.

Stallion – uncastrated older male pony.

Submission – yield without resistance, surrender.

Surcingle – strap that goes around the torso of the pony. Some hold on saddles, others are equipped for training purposes such as holding side reins in place.

Suspension – when the energy of the movement is more off the ground than not. The strides may seem shorter.

Tack – any of the various equipment and accessories worn by ponies. Saddles, stirrups, bridles, halters, reins, bits, harnesses, martingales and breastplates are all forms of horse tack. In the case of the human pony, it may include all or part of the costume.

Tacking up – the act of putting the costume, tack and/or equipment on the pony.

Tempi Changes – canter lead changes in numerical sets. It may start with four strides working down to three, two and one strides between changes.

Top – person who takes the role of the controller, in this case the trainer.

Trail riding – riding down the open road or cross-country.

Transition – moving from one gait to another.

Trot – a natural jogging gait with a moment of suspension between strides. In human pony play the trot is like the human jog.

Volt – a small circle – six meters in diameter.

Turn out – 1. to let a horse out for free exercise in an enclosure, 2. to groom and or dress the pony for the purpose of presentation and/or competition.

Walk – moving forward placing one foot firmly down upon the ground before picking up the next. Individual ponies vary in the smoothness of their walk. The fastest walk is the "running walk" of the Tennessee Walking Horse. If a horse begins to speed up and lose a regular cadence to its gait, the horse is no longer walking, but is beginning to either trot or move into an alternative ambling or "single foot" gait. In human pony play it is a two beat gait resembling a human walk, but can be developed as the trainer sees fit, such as in an extension or in the high-stepping often used in pony play.

Warm-blood – generally speaking, a cross-breed of a hot-blood and cold-blood pony. Warm-bloods tend to be athletic and even tempered.

Willing – "Willing" is the term used by equestrians to describe a horse that chooses to do what the trainer or handler asks of their own free will in a positive spirit of cooperation.

Appendix D
Related Resources

The Stampede

> http://www.the-stampede.com/

Pony Sites

> http://www.fetishpony.com/
> http://www.npony.com/
> http://www.chargerpony.com/main.html

Kinky Pony Girl

> http://www.kinkyponygirl.com

Pupett

> http://www.pupett.com/guest/ponygirl_eng.php

Trigger: The Human Equine

> http://www.thehumanequine.com/the1.html

Equus Eroticus Magazine

> http://www.equuseroticus.com/

Strawberry

> http://www.home.no/strawberryblonde/strawberryblonde.swf

Madonna

> http://www.madonnalicious.com/archive/may2006.html

The Other Pony Club

> http://www.tawse.com

The Other World Kingdom

http://www.owk.cz/index.htm

House of Gord

http://www.houseofgord.com/

JG Leathers

http://www.jg-leathers.com/

Article:

http://www.maximumawesome.com/pervfriday/ponypeople.htm

Deviant Desires

http://www.deviantdesires.com/map/mapmain.html

Dutch Pony

http://dutchpony.data-service.nl/

If you would like to learn more about speaking to horses try

http://www.horsewhisperer.com/ or http://www.montyroberts.com/

Gear

http://www.prodeviant.com

http://www.sub-shop.com/

http://www.water-hole.com/

http://www.marquis.de/onlineshop/

http://www.fantasyleather.co.uk/

http://www.huse.com/

http://www.reactor.net.au/

Books and Mags

Pony Play Manual, by Jessica Brown

http://www.tawse.com/

Equus Eroticus

http://www.equuseroticus.com/

Jay Wiseman's Erotic Bondage Handbook

http://www.greenerypress.com

The Klutz Book of Knots

http://www.klutz.com

Video

Andreas Helgstrand - WEG2006 Freestyle Final

http://www.youtube.com/watch?v=zKQgTiqhPbw

Patches the Coolest Horse

http://www.youtube.com/watch?v=teHfyby_veU

Documentary: **Born in a Barn**

http://www.threegracesfilms.com/projects.html

Fox Hunt excerpt

http://www.sextelevision.net/archives/episodeArchivesDisplay.
asp?episodeID=198&segmentID=518&seasonID=9

Pony Girl Prancing (At Burningman)

http://www.youtube.com/watch?v=baFzLOfodWI&feature=related

Pony Girl 5

http://www.youtube.com/watch?v=3Hz6X214xU4&feature=related

Ponygirl Rose

http://www.youtube.com/watch?v=1ByIOh4z1HQ&feature=related

Networking

http://groups.yahoo.com/group/ponyplayersunited/

http://groups.yahoo.com/group/StampedeTalk/

http://groups.yahoo.com/group/Other_Pony_Club/?yguid=290755725

http://ponyplay.tribe.net/

http://ponygirlsnboys.tribe.net/

Photography

http://www.luvbight.com/

http://www.darlingpropaganda.com/

http://www.jumbobrain.com - Mike Woolson

Etcetera:

Ponymistress Rebecca

http://www.myspace.com/ponymistress

Acknowledgments _____

The pony community from around the world contributed to this endeavor in hopes to make the world a little smaller for ponies. It is but a tip of the iceberg for all that is pony. Thank you.

Special thanks to the two ponies who carried this book. Pupett of www.pupett.com, who owes me a pony date, thank you for your generosity and support through this project. Your deep love of the "naughty" pony makes me laugh and brings such depth to the book. Penny Barber of www.PennyBarber.com, my little filly, Copper, who's so willing, thank you for putting up with the hours and hours of photos that were more work than play. I promise to work less and play more. That goes for the photographer, my partner, The Monkey, too.

Thank you for supporting me and this project to the end. To all those who gave of their hearts and lives to be both in the book and the support crew behind the book, thank you, you made this book what it is – beautiful.

With sincere gratitude,
Rebecca Wilcox, Ponymistress

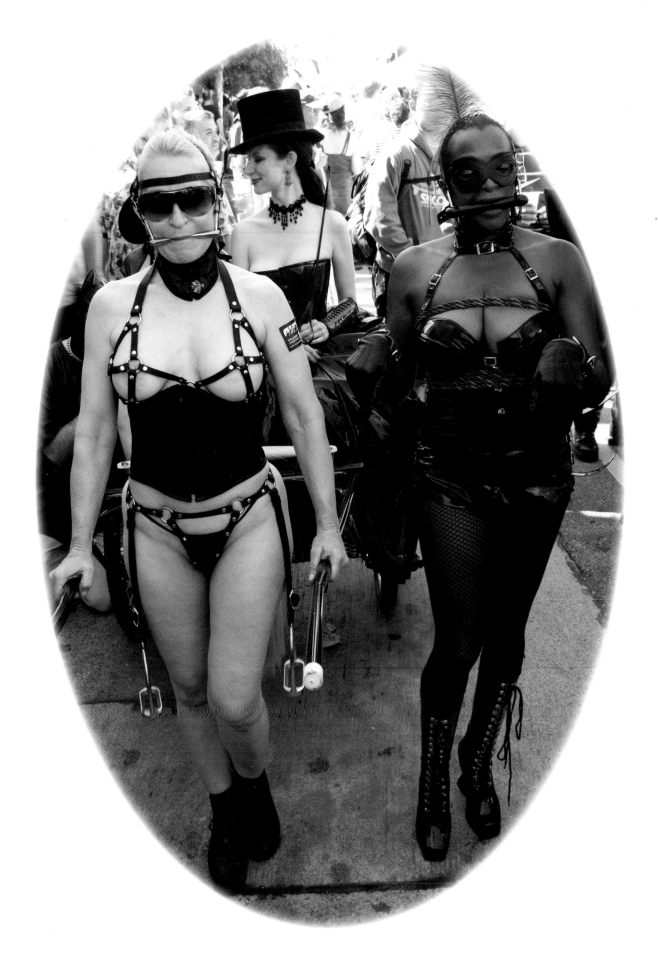

Photograph by Mark Burnley, "Folsom Street Fair" — © www.seriousbondage.com.